THAI MASSAGE

THAI MASSAGE

Knowing Where and How to Touch

Beatrice Avraham

Astrolog ◆ The Quality of Life Series ◆

Series editor: Sara Bleich
Editor: Marion Duman
Cover design: Na'ama Yaffe
Layout and Graphics: Ruth Erez
Production Manager: Dan Gold
Photographs applied by the author.

ISBN 965-494-117-1

Published by Astrolog Publishing House 2001

Astrolog Publishing House

P. O. Box 1123, Hod Hasharon 45111, Israel
Tel: 972-9-7412044
Fax: 972-9-7442714
E-Mail: info@astrolog.co.il

Printed in Israel

1 3 5 7 9 10 8 6 4 2

Thanks

With deep feelings of love and pride, I thank my three children for their unconditional support in the fulfillment of my dreams, and for their practical contribution - more valuable than any treasure - to their realization.

I would like to express my appreciation to my loyal secretary, Rachel, who shared all the deliberations involved in the writing of this book.

My love and thanks go to several true friends, upon whose bodies I learned to apply the secret of Thai magic.

I would like to thank my good friend, Mashi Zarfati, whose photograph appears on the cover of this book.

Contents

INTRODUCTION

The original name of Thai massage is "Nuad Thai." In Thailand and in many Asiatic countries, people who suffer from problems concerning their physical functioning are not considered "ill" in the Western sense of the term, but rather as people whose personal equilibrium - either on the mental or the physical plane - has been temporarily upset. For this reason, they receive holistic treatment, with the aim of restoring equilibrium to all the body's elements.

The birth of Thai massage is linked to the name of a physician from northern India, who lived 2,500 years ago, and to the strong friendship between him and Buddha. Jivaka Kumar Bhaccha was a contemporary of Buddha, and in Thailand, his name gradually became Shivago Komarpaj. The renowned center for Thai massage is named in his memory: The Foundation of Shivago Komarpaj, Traditional Buntautuk Hospital, Chiang Mai, Thailand.

This great man is the source of the basic knowledge of today's massage techniques, as well as of the healing powers of various plants, steam, yoga, and minerals, which, together with the well-known methods of Chinese medicine, constituted the entity called "traditional-alternative medicine."

Thai massage belongs to this entity, and is founded on the premise that the human body contains a large number of invisible energy lines (about 72,000 in all) that are called "sens."

In Thai massage, the sens are the same as the meridians in the Chinese arts of acupuncture and acupressure, and in the Japanese art of Shiatsu.

It is commonly thought that Thai massage originated in the Indian tradition (and in fact, some of the Indian names have been preserved). Life energy, called "prana," is absorbed into the body from the air and food, via the processes of breathing and digestion (according to the theory of Indian philosophy).

The energy lines (ten of which are considered crucially important) are invisible, and they constitute a perfect system, close to the human body. In the Indian language, the "prana nadis" are the sens, and this system is like a "second body" that is called "pranamaya kosha" or "the body's energy."

Thai massage is applied to the treatment points (acupressure points) that are situated along the ten central energy lines. Its aim is therapeutic. Its basic premise states that diseases or disturbances in health are caused by blockages in the flow of the energy in the body. By means of massage, the unimpaired flow is restored, as is equilibrium.

Massage is not performed for profit, but rather is considered a spiritual aid that is offered to a person who is suffering, and generally accompanies the study of Buddhism. For many years, practical studies took place in the framework of monasteries (Wat Pho in Bangkok is one of the most important), and the masseurs linked their work to the application of Buddhism. The masseur generally begins his work with prayer and deep concentration, enabling him to focus on the patient. (Traditionally, the recipient of the treatment is called a patient, even though he may not be ill.) The practitioner, who is in a meditative state, hones his senses toward the energy lines and the treatment points, toward problems that require treatment, and toward the sensitivity of every patient.

Thai massage does not resemble Western massage techniques (except for reflexology, which is slightly reminiscent of it), and is divided into two types:

1. General massage for a good feeling, a feeling of relief, flexibility, and energetic balance.
2. Therapeutic massage for alleviating various medical problems; this type is practiced only by highly experienced, qualified practitioners.

It must be remembered that massage is not a game, although it is supposed to be a means of providing pleasure for patient and practitioner alike. It is highly recommended that people who intend working in this field - even in the general type of massage, not the therapeutic kind - undergo basic training in order to be beneficial and not cause damage.

The beginner practitioner must gradually hone his senses toward other people's bodies, since no two people are alike, and the massage must suit the individual body structure of each patient.

As each person reacts differently to each massage technique, the practitioner regulates the strength of the pressure, the tension, and so on, so that the treatment will give the patient an overall good feeling, without suffering.

General body massage requires between two and two and a half hours, and must be done slowly, with deep concentration, and without repeating the exercises. When the practitioner has less time than this available, he should limit the massage to part of the body only, and perform a complete massage on it. There are hundreds of possible exercises for each region of the body, and the practitioner selects them according to the nature, problems, and needs of the patient.

In the first part of the book, 135 exercises are presented, from which the practitioner selects the ones that suit the patient's needs. The practitioner chooses a number of exercises for every part of the body. There is always a set order for them - 1 to 135; he does not go backward, and performs only the selected exercises, in order.

In the second part, which is meant for self-massage, 77 exercises are presented. If the person has a specific problem, he need perform only the particular set of exercises relevant to that problem or to that body part, or to various body parts that affect the problem, according to the order of the exercises. If the person is performing the massage in order to prevent problems, he must do all the exercises in order - 1 to 77. However, he can omit exercises that require particular exertion or pliancy that he lacks.

The sitting position of the practitioner is a function of the experience he has accumulated. Over time, he learns what the most comfortable position for performing each exercise is. The basic principle in the choice of exercises is going from easy to difficult, from the simple ones to the more complicated ones, in order to get the patient's body gradually accustomed to the various procedures.

During the treatment, it is a very good idea to have soft, relaxing music playing in the background. Moreover, the patient is fully dressed in light, comfortable clothes.

There are several trends in Thai massage, the most important of which are the "Northern Method" and the "Southern Method." This book is based on the Northern Method, which is taught in the Foundation of Shivago Komarpaj Medical Complex in Chiang Mai, Northern Thailand.

The Composition of the Human Being

The human being is made up of the four elements of nature:

1. Earth
2. Water
3. Wind
4. Fire

Every part of the human being represents one of the elements, and there must be equilibrium between them.

The parallels between the elements and the human being are:

Earth - the structure, build of the human being, all the organs.
Water - the fluids that flow in the body, such as blood, lymph, fat.
Wind - the movement of the human being, every part that moves in his body.
Fire - energy, body temperature, digestion processes.

When the four elements are in harmony, the person is healthy, and there is equilibrium between all of his body parts and their functions. If there is a lack or an excess of the elements, the situation is abnormal, and leads to diseases. In a case such as this, the treatment will begin with an attempt to bring the elements into balance, and to this end, physiotherapy, meditation, massage, sauna, and so on, are used.

Energy lines and treatment points on the various parts of the body

The energy lines of the leg

a. The outer side of the leg.
b. The inner side of the leg.

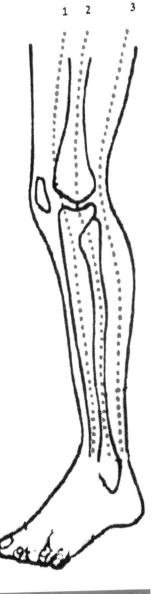

On the outer side of the leg, there are three energy lines:

Line number 1 passes behind the tibia in the lower part of the leg and continues upward. In the region of the knee, the line begins on the outermost border of the kneecap, and runs behind the thigh.

Line number 2 begins in the lower part of the leg, in the upper ankle region above the protruding ankle bone, at the upper end of the fibula, and continues upward. In the region of the knee, the beginning of the line can be located in the hollow at the side of the knee.

Line number 3 can be identified and worked on most easily when the person is lying on his side. It begins in the lower part of the leg near the Achilles tendon, and continues along the tendon, between the tendon and the bone. In the region of the knee, it begins at the upper end of the tendon, the side, and the knee, and continues straight in the direction of the tendon. The continuation of the line passes the buttocks, and reaches the pelvis.

On the inner side of the leg, there are three energy lines:

Line number 1 on the lower part of the leg runs exactly behind the tibia and continues upward. At the knee, the line begins behind the outer border of the kneecap and continues straight to the groin.

Line number 2 on the lower part of the leg is located in the hollow at the side of the protruding ankle bone. In the region of the knee, there is another hollow (at the side of the knee), and this point indicates the beginning of an energy line that then goes straight to the groin.

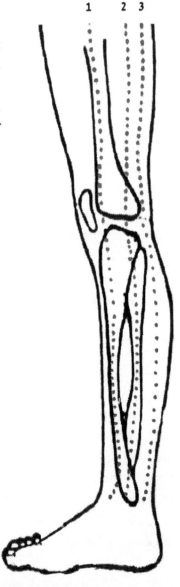

Line number 3 on the lower part of the leg runs from the Achilles heel along the back of the curve of the heel. In the region of the knee, it is possible to feel a tendon joint, and the massage is performed above the tendon in the direction of the groin.

Treatment points

On the foot there are extremely important treatment points:

Point 1 is located exactly below the ankle. This point is very sensitive, and is connected to the sexual system. It is a therapeutic point for problems concerning this system (menstrual problems and impotence).

Point 2 is used for relaxation, and the application of pressure to it indirectly affects point 1.

(These two points **must not** be worked on in pregnant women.)

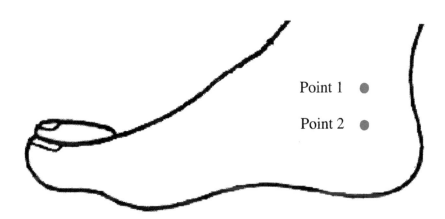

The sole of the foot - massage and pressure points

On the sole of the foot, there are several treatment points that are connected to various parts of the body, and affect the functioning of those parts.

On the **inner** side of the foot, the points are **different** on each foot. In order to affect the functioning of a certain part of the body, and improve it, the appropriate points on the foot must be worked, and pressures and turning movements applied.

There are at least two different ways to perform the massage of the sole of the foot: The first one is to start the massage at the center point on the heel (inner side - point A) and apply thumb pressures in the direction of the toes - in this way, most of the treatment points of the sole of the foot are included, and damage is avoided. The second way is to begin the pressures from five points along a common line on the inner side of the heel, and continue the massage up to the tips of the toes (the line marked X-X).

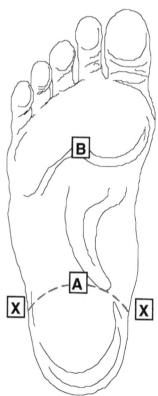

The upper surface of the foot

On the upper surface of the foot, the massage starts from the point where the toe bones join the lower leg - point C. Thumb pressures are not applied, but rather turning movements between the tendons that separate the toes, to their tips, and finally pressure must be applied to the pads of the toes. The thumbs perform the turning movements: at first, one thumb is placed on top of the other while applying pressure to point C; then the length of the tendons on every pair of toes (the middle toe does not have a partner) must be massaged by rotation movements. Finally, each toe is pulled outward separately, while the foot is held in one hand, and the toe is pulled by two fingers of the practitioner's other hand. (The massage methods will be discussed later.)

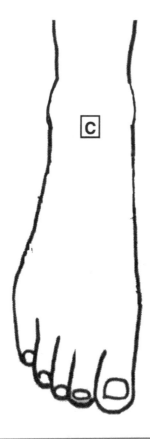

The connecting muscle

On the sole of the foot, there is a connecting muscle, and on it there are five treatment points to which pressure must be applied by the thumbs. This can be done when both feet are being massaged simultaneously, or during the massage of each foot separately.

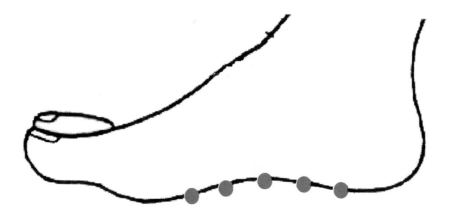

Treatment points of the leg - acupressure
for cases of lower back pains (in particular)

Pressure is applied three times to each point: weak, medium, strong. The pressure should be applied on both feet simultaneously, using the thumbs.

Of course, pressure should be applied only **after** the application of palm pressure (P.P.), thumb pressure (T.P.) up to the knees and behind them, along the inner and outer energy lines (on each leg separately), and the stretching of the legs (each leg separately). (This will be discussed later.)

At the end of the treatment, Walking P.P. must be applied to both legs simultaneously.

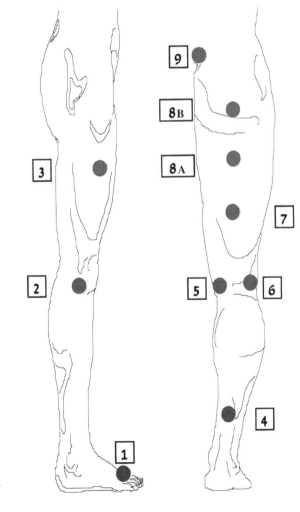

Treatment points of the thigh

In the region of the thigh bone, there are three treatment points: The first is very close to the hollow that is next to the bone, and the two others are lower, on each side of the first point (see diagram). These are the treatment points of the outer thigh, upon which the pressures are mainly turning, using the thumbs and palms (to be discussed).

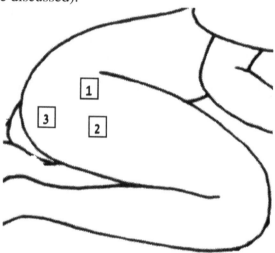

In the region of the inner thigh, starting from the thigh bone toward the kneecap, there are three treatment points close to one another. Massage in this region is performed by the soles of the feet, which will be described in foot massage later on.

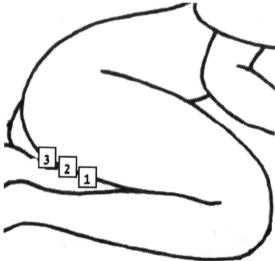

Treatment points and energy lines of the hand and palm

Point 1 is known by the name "Hegu" in acupuncture, and it is a very important point. Applying pressure to this point alleviates every kind of pain: head, stomach, teeth, facial paralysis, cold. The pressures cause strong local pain, but this pain brings relief. (This is forbidden for pregnant women.)

Points 2 and 3 are recommended for headaches and toothache.

Point 4 is recommended for problems of knee pains and sciatica.

Point 5 is recommended for sore throats and toothache.

Point 6 is recommended for a stiff neck.

Point 7 is recommended for shoulder pains and pains in the bone joints.

Point 8 is recommended for pains in the neck, shoulders, arms, and hands, and for stomach-aches and migraines.

Point 9 is recommended for nausea and vertigo.

Point 10 is recommended for shortness of breath, pains in the chest, back, and shoulders, and wrist diseases.

Point 11 is recommended for wrist diseases and hand paralysis.

Point 12 is recommended for insomnia and angina pectoris.

Point 13 is recommended for coughs, asthma, fever, sore throats, and tendon diseases.

Point 14 is recommended for sore throats, respiratory problems, and fever.

Point 15 is recommended for whooping cough and arthritis of the hands.

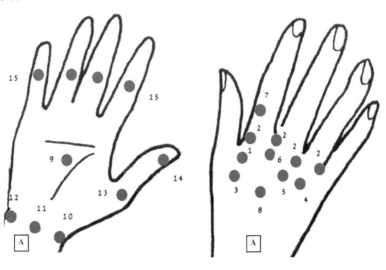

The energy lines of the arm

Although there are several energy lines on the arm, it is customary to massage two inner energy lines and one outer energy line.

The inner energy lines start at the wrist and run in the direction of the elbow. They continue below and above the front side of the biceps toward the armpit. (Care must be taken not to apply pressure to bones.)

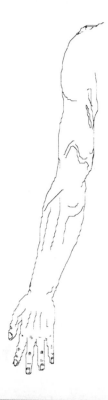

The outer energy line starts at the wrist and runs to the shoulder, along the whole arm, following the central and separating line between the two upper muscles.

The energy lines of the back

The two energy lines of the back run along each side of the spinal column. The first line is located at a distance of a finger-width from the spine, and the second is located at a distance of a finger-width from the first line. They are especially effective for treating stomach, spleen, pancreas, and kidney problems, and of course for shoulder, neck, and back pains.

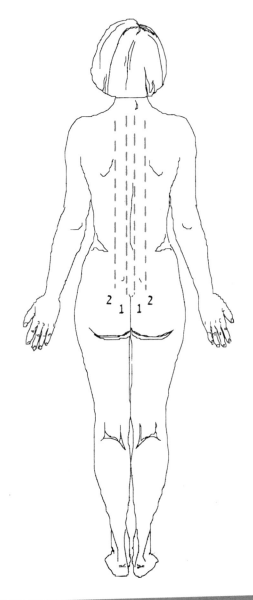

Treating the energy lines of the back is very effect in most problems of the functioning of the body. Massage in this case cannot cause damage, and it should be performed several times.

In the region of the shoulders and nape, there are three treatment points (massage by P.P., T.P., elbow pressure, sliding the forearm - to be discussed later.)

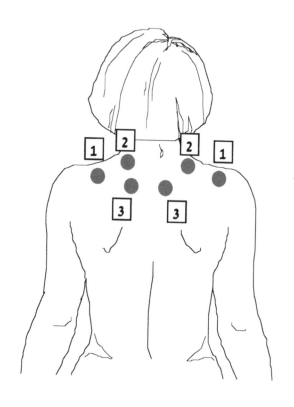

Treatment points on the abdomen (by pressure)

Massage is generally performed in a clockwise direction. (Note: In cases of constipation, the massage of the points is performed in a **clockwise** direction; in cases of diarrhea, the massage of the points is performed in an **anti-clockwise** direction.)

Point 1 is the central point - the navel - which is also the center of the all the body's energy lines.

Points 2, 3 are located at a distance of a finger from the navel. These must be worked on twice.

Points A, B are special treatment points in cases of hernia, abnormal periods, and excessive menstrual bleeding.

Points 1/13 - navel and intestines.

Points 10, 9, 7, 2/8 - intestines.

Point 3 - stomach.

Point 4 - liver.

Points 11, 6 - kidneys.

Point 12 - stomach and spleen.

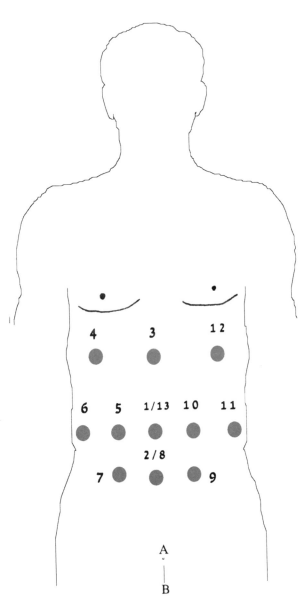

Energy lines on the abdomen

Lines 1, 2 are located on each side of the navel. The fingers press by massage next to the navel, at a distance of a finger from the navel line (N).

Lines 3, 4 run along the front of the body, close to the sides. The fingers massage by pressures below the bands of muscles.

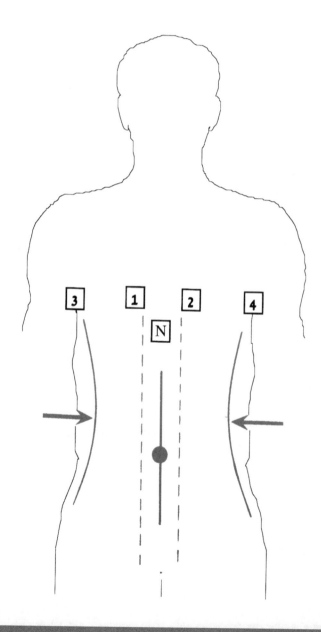

Treatment points on the head and face

The head has a central line, which begins at point 1, which is located in the hollow at the base of the skull, and traverses the head until it reaches point 2. Along this line, there are numerous treatment points, very close to one another. Massage is performed with T.P., thumb on thumb, starting from point number 1, up to point number 2, which is located at the beginning of the forehead. (This is also the weekly routine in yoga.) The rest of the massage consists of turning movements.

Pair of points 3 is located on each side of the hollow at the base of the skull. They are extremely sensitive to pressure, and it is very easy to locate them. Massaging these points is very effective in cases of headaches. In a general massage, they can be omitted.

Pair of points 4, 5, 6 are located in the hollows behind the ears. Massage is performed by the thumbs, using turning movements, light pressures only.

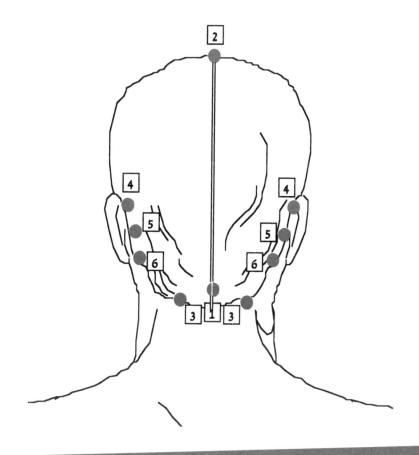

The face

The treatment points on the face are numerous, and energy lines run between them. The massage of the face includes applying pressure to specific points as well as massage by the palms toward the energy lines (circular massage), from the direction of the chin toward the forehead.

Point 1 - "the third eye" - is an extremely important point, and is considered the sixth most important energy center in the human body (out of seven centers).

Point 2 - a treatment point for headaches, insomnia, and sinusitis.

Points 3, 4, 5, 6 - treatment points for headaches and facial paralysis.

Points 7 - on the temples, extremely important treatment points for headaches, migraines, and facial paralysis.

Points 8 - at the beginning of the tear ducts, treatment points for insomnia. Pressure is applied for up to a minute, several times (T.P.).

Points 9, 10, 11 - located in the little hollows next to the ears. Massage is a therapy in cases of earache, toothache, and deafness.

Points 12 - the treatment points in cases of sinusitis and facial paralysis.

Point 13 - the "unconscious" point. It is very important for treating cases of weakness, fainting, shock, sunstroke, and respiratory defects.

Point 14 - a treatment point in cases of facial paralysis.

Points 15 - treatment points in cases of migraines.

Comment: The massage of the head and face is extremely important, even if there is no need to treat specific problems. Massage induces relaxation, releases tension, and dispels fatigue.

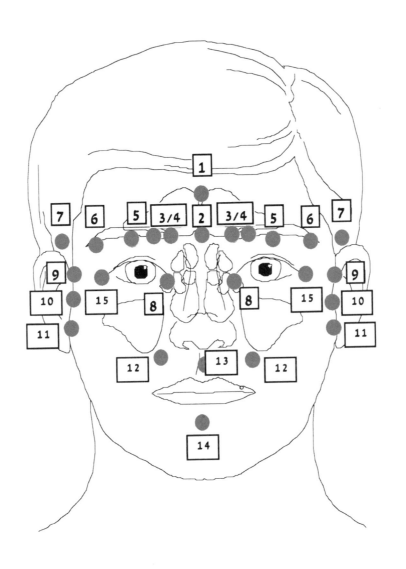

The theoretical basis for Thai massage: The ten energy lines (Ten Sen)

The meridians in China, the "prana nadis" in yoga, the "chakras" in yoga, and the "sens" in Thailand are based on ancient cumulative experience. Their common denominator is that the "method" works very well. The energy lines are not an anatomical fact, and cannot be identified. They are, in effect, channels for the flow of energy in the human body.

The practitioner utilizes knowledge for performing the massage, and he acquires this knowledge mainly through experience.

Therapeutic treatments are based - unequivocally - on the massage of a particular energy line, as will be described later on.

All the energy lines begin at the navel, which is the body's energetic center.

1. Sen Sumana

Starts at the navel, passes through the chest cavity and the esophagus up to the tip of the tongue. It is identical to Sushumana Nadi in yoga and the Ren Mai meridian in Chinese acupuncture.

Massage: Abdomen, solar plexus, back, acupressure.

Therapy: Asthma, bronchitis, heart diseases, stomach and chest cramps, nausea, colds, coughs, digestive problems.

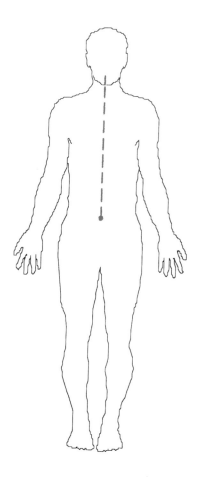

2. Sen Ittha

Starts on the left side of the navel, descends along the first outer energy line of the left leg, turns around the knee, and ascends along outer energy line number 3 of the left leg, runs along the left side of the spinal column, reaches the crown of the head (via the nape), and descends to the left nostril. It is identical to the Ida Nadi in yoga.

Massage: Full massage, legs, abdomen, back, shoulders, nape.

Therapy: Coughs, nasal blockages, respiratory problems, eye pains, fever, intestinal problems, back pains, bladder diseases, knee problems.

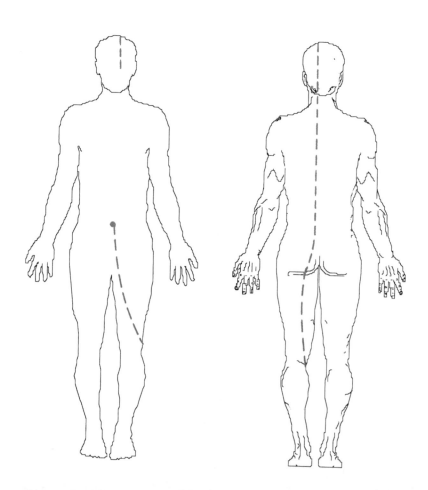

3. Sen Pingkhala

This energy line is located on the other side of the body relative to Sen Ittha, and is symmetrical to it, on the right side of the body. It is identical to the Pingala Nadi in yoga.

Massage: As in number 2.

Therapy: Similar to Sen Ittha, with the addition of liver and gall-bladder diseases.

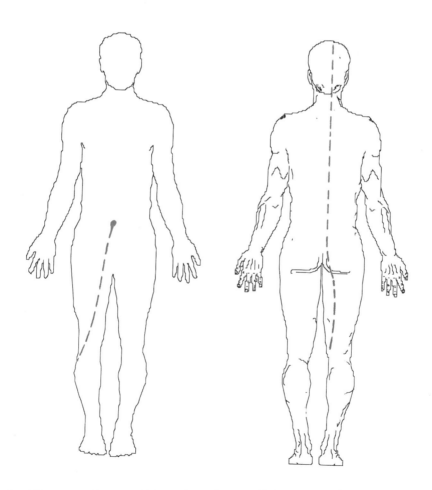

4. Sen Kalathari (four branches)

Starts at the navel and divides into two branches on the left side of the body and two on the right.

A. From the navel, it runs through the chest cavity and the shoulders, through the center line of the inner arm to the end of the hand, and from here to the fingertips (on both sides of the body).

B. From the navel, it runs downward via the central line of the inner leg to the foot, and from here to the tips of the toes (on both sides of the body).

Massage: P.P., T.P., P.P., (see further on) blood stopping, acupressure.

Therapy: Digestive problems, hernia, paralysis of the arms or legs, knee pains, arthritis, chest pains, heart problems linked to rheumatism, irregular heartbeat, blood flow problems, sinusitis, pains in the arms and legs, angina pectoris, epilepsy, mental diseases, mental disturbances.

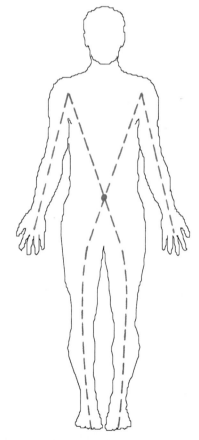

5. Sen Sahatsarangsi

Starts at the navel and runs along the first inner energy line of the left leg, continues along the first outer energy line, through the abdomen, the chest cavity, and the head, to the left eye. It is identical to the stomach meridian in China.

Massage: Massage of the leg (first inner and second outer energy lines), facial massage, acupressure.

Therapy: Facial paralysis, inflammations of the teeth, esophagus problems, fever, chest pains, psychoses and depressions, arthritis of the knee, thigh pains, eye problems.

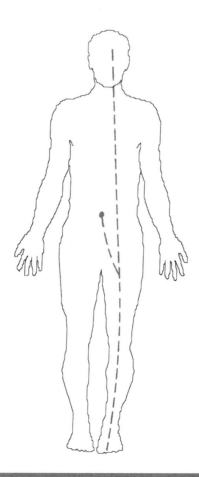

6. Sen Thawari

Identical to number 5 and symmetrical to it, on the right side of the body.

Massage: The same as number 5, on the right side.

Therapy: Similar to number 5, with the addition of appendicitis.

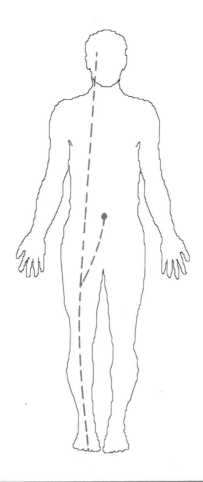

7. Sen Lawusang

Starts at the navel, runs through the solar plexus, the chest cavity, the left breast, to the left ear.

Massage: Massage of the shoulders, nape, face, acupressure.

Therapy: Ear diseases, coughs, facial paralysis, teeth problems, chest pains, digestive diseases.

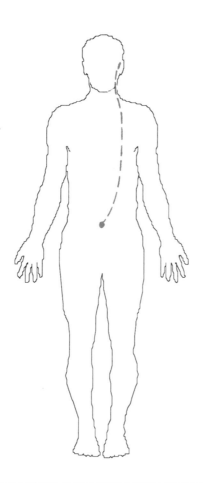

8. Sen Ulangka (Sen Rucham)

Similar to number 7, but on the right side of the body.

Massage: The same as number 7, on the right side.

Therapy: The same as number 7.

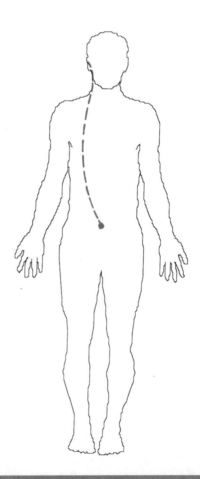

9. Sen Nanthakrawat

It consists of two energy lines:

One begins at the navel and runs to the bladder (Sen Sikhini).

The other begins at the navel and runs to the anus (Sen Sukhumang).

Massage: Massage of the abdomen in a clockwise direction in cases of constipation, and anti-clockwise in cases of diarrhea. P.P. with the pads of the fingers ("upright" palm). The fingers apply pressure to the treatment points (7 points). (See further on.)

Therapy: In order to affect it, the stomach (abdomen) is massaged. It is used for treating cases of hernias, and fertility problems:

In women - the bladder, irregular periods.

In men - impotence, premature ejaculation, diarrhea, abdominal pains.

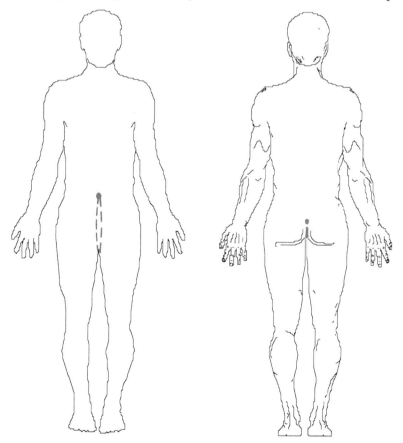

10. Sen Khitchanna

Similar to number 9. Runs from the navel to the male genitals (Sen Pitakun), or from the navel to the female genitals (Sen Kitcha).

Massage: Massage of the abdomen and perineum.

Therapy: Massaging the abdomen affects it. It is used for treating problems similar to the ones in number 9.

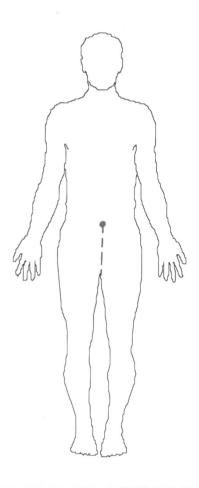

Guidelines for the Practitioner

1. Before the massage

The first stage before performing the massage is a conversation with the patient in order to clarify his state of health: diseases, operations, blood pressure, pregnancy, hernias, diseases of the blood vessels, stomach or intestinal problems, constipation, diarrhea, lower or upper back problems.

Before beginning the treatment, the patient and the practitioner wash their hands and feet in order to eliminate negative energies.

2. Rules for the massage

Sores must not be touched. Bones, the spinal column, knees, and elbows must not be massaged.

In cases of high blood pressure or blood-vessel problems, the exercises for blood stopping in the arms and legs must not be performed.

In cases of stomach or intestinal problems, the abdomen must not be massaged.

The knees are the most sensitive focal point, and must be related to with extreme caution during treatment. They must not be massaged directly.

Acupressure must not be performed on very tired muscles or in places where there are muscle cramps. Pressure must not be applied to the lymph glands.

Patients with heart diseases must consult their physician before undergoing a massage. In general, they can undergo light stretching and head and face massage.

Pregnant women must not undergo massage, except on the energy lines of the legs, arms and back (when seated), and on the head and face.

All the exercises marked with an asterisk (∗) should be performed only by people who have the necessary qualifications and experience, and in accordance with the specific limitations.

Work rules for the practitioner

You must work in a quiet, calm atmosphere, with maximum concentration. You must begin the consultation with a conversation with the patient about his state of health and inquire about any diseases and operations.

Work gently, not with force.

Before and after the massage of any body part, apply turning hand pressures for relaxation (P.P.) and work in a turning manner with the thumbs after applying the pressure (T.P.) to any point. (See Methods of Treatment, further on.)

Work with straight arms and a straight back, with the strength of the pressure applied stemming from the weight of the entire body.

When using thumb pressures (T.P.), use the pads of the fingers, and not the fingertips or the nails.

Abdominal massage must not be performed sooner than three hours after a meal.

Massage of men begins on the right side of the body, while massage of women begins on the left side of the body. During an abdominal massage, women's knees are bent, while men's legs are straight.

In the East, it is customary to begin the treatment with prayer, which enables the participants to enter a state of maximum concentration.

Massage is an exchange of energies between practitioner and patient, in an attempt to restore the patient's equilibrium.

When the patient's body is full of negative energies, the practitioner takes them upon himself, and he feels tired and even ill. It is therefore very important that the practitioner perform meditation and relaxation exercises after the treatment, in order to restore his own equilibrium. Moreover, he must wash his hands thoroughly at the end of the treatment so as to eliminate the negative energies he has received.

The techniques that are recommended here are for healthy people, not for healing purposes. A practitioner who does not have the appropriate qualifications must not undertake to administer therapeutic treatment.

Massage is part of a set of life habits that include correct nutrition, a positive attitude toward life, giving and receiving love in all its forms, optimism, self-love, and love of others.

The exercises that are described in this book are mainly meant for couples, so that each member of the couple can perform them on the other.

A suitable atmosphere of relaxation should be created by means of soft music, a comfortable room temperature, and a room that is as quiet as possible (get the children out, turn off phones, cell-phones, etc.).

Thai massage does not utilize oils, because during the pressures, the fingers slip on oily skin. However, at the end of the treatment, it is possible to sprinkle a few drops of almond oil on the patient's body, and massage it by light stroking movements.

Frequently, the patient falls asleep during the treatment, and this is a true indication of relaxation and a successful massage. It is not real sleep, but rather a state of "between dream and reality," which many people especially enjoy.

The perfect results of the massage are visible and felt properly about 48 hours after the treatment. The good feeling in the body is felt immediately.

The exercises must be performed one after the other, without interruption.

Methods of work - treatment

The methods of work are presented in order of their occurrence in the exercises. After reading the introduction, you are advised to look at the photographs of the various exercises, and see how each massage method is actually performed.

1. Palm pressure - P.P.

Pressure is applied with the palms along the energy lines; the arms are kept straight. The pressure stems from the weight of the entire body, which moves from side to side together with the hand that is applying the pressure.

P.P. is performed at the beginning and end of every massage. It is very helpful in relaxation, and can be performed back and forth several times.

In the region of the knees, turning movements are performed; pressure is not applied.

2. Thumb pressure - T.P.

Pressure is applied using the pad of one thumb along one of the energy lines, and the other thumb very close to the first, preparing to apply pressure.

When the second thumb begins to apply pressure, the first reduces the pressure, so that in fact the pressure alternates, back and forth, along the whole energy line.

Massage of the arms and legs is performed first on the inner part and then on the outer part.

3. Walking

This massage is performed both by the hands during P.P. and by the feet (while massaging the back, the abdomen, or the inner or outer side of the thighs).

Walking P.P. is applied when one hand applies pressure and the other is relaxed in the air, and vice versa.

4. Rotate (rotation) massage

This is performed mainly by the palms, when massaging the sole of the foot and the palm.

5. Circle massage

This is performed on the sole of the foot and on the shoulders, using the elbow.

6. Stretching

Stretching the leg is performed when one of the practitioner's hands holds the patient's leg at the groin, while his other hand holds the knee region, and he pulls in opposite directions (stretching the upper half of the leg - the thigh).

When stretching the whole leg, the practitioner's other hand holds the patient's leg in the region above the ankle, and he pulls in opposite directions.

Stretching the arm is performed by holding the patient's arm by the armpit in one hand, while the other holds the arm just above the elbow, and pulling in opposite directions.

7. Blood stopping

This action is performed on legs/arms.

It begins by the application of P.P. simultaneously on both legs (it can also be applied separately), back and forth. When the blood flow in the join between the leg and the groin is felt, the practitioner applies P.P. with the entire weight of his body (for up to 50 seconds), without moving.

If the patient experiences difficulty with this position, the pressure must be gradually reduced.

This exercise of stopping the blood is also performed on the arms, using both palms in the patient's armpits. After performing P.P., the practitioner applies pressure simultaneously with both palms along the patient's arm, from the elbow to the armpit.

Comment: These exercises are forbidden for people with cardiac diseases, high blood pressure, and blood-vessel diseases.

8. Squeezing

Squeezing (as with a wet towel) is performed with both hands "squeezing" the muscle in opposite directions.

9. P.P., T.P. with interlaced fingers

This massage is performed mainly on the nape, with P.P. applied by the pads of the hands, and the T.P. applied by the thumbs.

10. Chopping

This massage is performed with both hands together rapidly striking the patient's shoulders or back.

11. Sliding

This massage involves stroking the hand, foot, back, and so on.

12. Shaking

This is performed mainly at the end of the massage of the arms, as well as of the thighs.

13. Acupressure

When massaging the abdomen and the chest cavity, the practitioner applies pressures with the pads of three fingers: the second, third, and fourth.

14. Acupressure by thumb pressure

There are treatment points on the hand, the foot, the leg, the back, the face and the head. The practitioner uses the technique of applying pressure to specific points by one thumb after the other, or with one thumb (depending on the particular case) for five seconds, and turning movements in the same place with the same thumb/thumbs.

15. Twisting

This is performed on the arms, legs, and back, with both palms outstretched and applying pressure in opposite directions, without stretching.

16. Hitting

This massage is for balancing the muscles. It is performed with a fist along the part that is being worked on.

17. Spinal Twist

The practitioner performs "squeezing" with his hands on one side of the patient's back, and afterwards turns the patient onto his other side and repeats the massage.

The squeezing movements are performed using the fingers and palms, back and forth on the back.

18. Shampooing

This massage resembles shampooing one's head, and is performed at the end of the head massage, using the pads of the fingers of both hands.

MASSAGE EXERCISES 1-135

Basic massage stages

Warming and relaxing by applying palm pressure with the palms of the hands back and forth several times (P.P.)

Applying thumb pressure (T.P.) along the energy lines.

Relaxing by applying palm pressure (P.P.).

Stretching.

Blood stopping in the arm and the leg in cases in which the patient does not suffer from heart problems, blood pressure, and blood-vessel diseases.

Massage serves two purposes: relaxation and therapy, and by means of the method, pressure is applied to help the flow of energy.

Before treatment, it is advisable to use steam - such as in a sauna - so as to increase the energy flow.

Massaging legs and feet (Ex. 1-42)

Exercise 1

The patient lies on his back with his legs open.
The practitioner kneels, with his buttocks resting on his feet.
The practitioner's two hands massage the patient's two feet alternately;
the practitioner leans to the left and to the right, in the direction of the
hand that is applying the pressure.

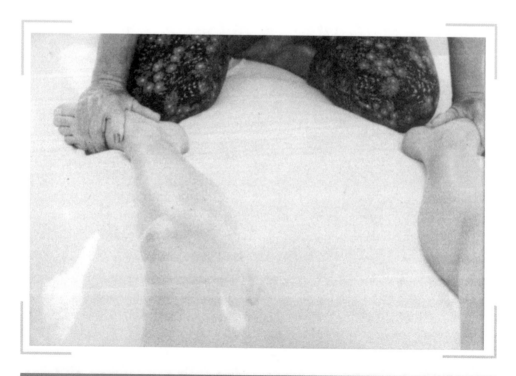

Exercise 2

The patient is in the same position.
The practitioner uses open hands to massage the patient's legs in the direction of the knees, moving alternately right and left, back and forth.

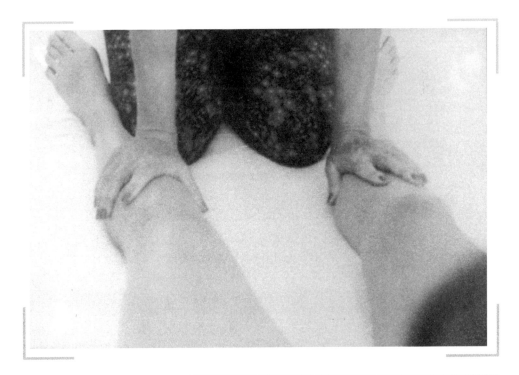

Exercise 3

The patient is in the same position.
The practitioner uses his palms to massage the patient's knees with rotation movements in both directions, several times.

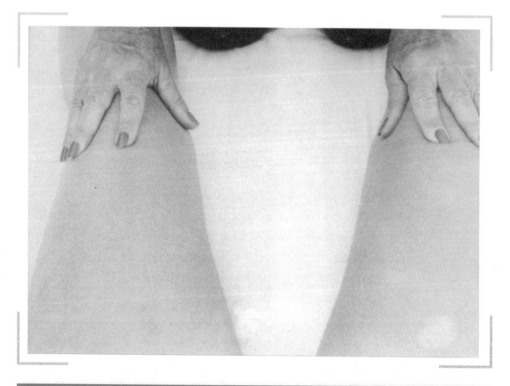

Exercise 4

The patient lies on his back, his ankles downward, and his toes upward.
The practitioner sits in a comfortable position.
On the foot, there are a number of points to which T.P. must be applied
(see the diagram of the foot in the Introduction) to the same points
simultaneously on both feet. Pressure is applied three times to each pair
of points, for five seconds each time.

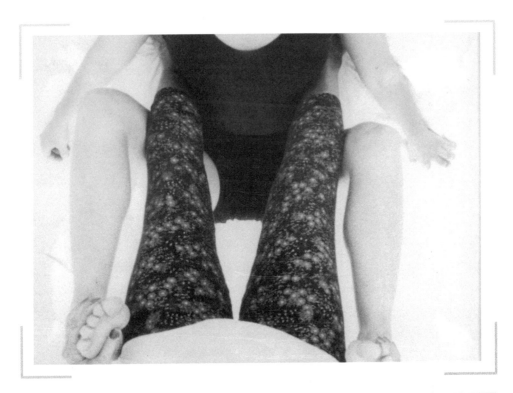

Exercise 5

The patient is in the same position.
The practitioner kneels.
The practitioner begins the massage of the foot using both thumbs, with the patient's ankle resting on his knee.
Rotate massage is performed from the toes toward the ankle and back.
At the end of the exercise, for relaxation: light palm drumming on the upper surface of the foot.

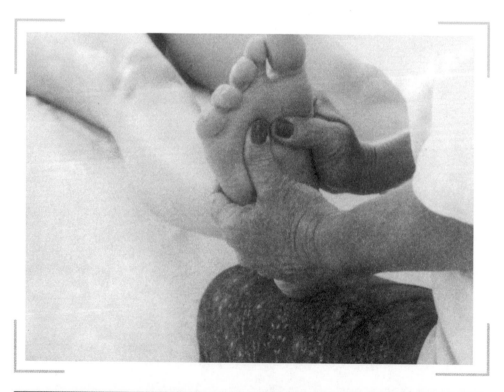

Exercise 6

The patient and the practitioner are in the same position.
On the inner side of the foot, there is a muscle that joins the sole to the
upper surface of the foot. There are five treatment points on this muscle
(see the diagram in the Introduction). Pressure is applied using both
thumbs, from the ankle toward the toes and back, several times.

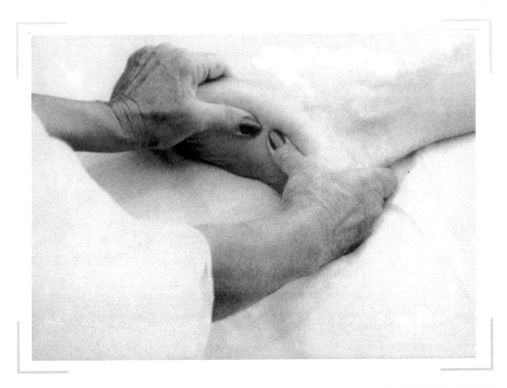

Exercise 7

The patient and the practitioner are in the same position.
The practitioner lifts the patient's foot and holds the toes from the
direction of upper surface of the foot in one hand, while he holds the
ankle in the other. The leg that is being worked on is supported in the
area of the calf by the practitioner's knees at an angle
that is comfortable for both.
At this point, the practitioner performs rotate massage on the patient's
foot three times in each direction, the active hand being
the one that is holding the toes.

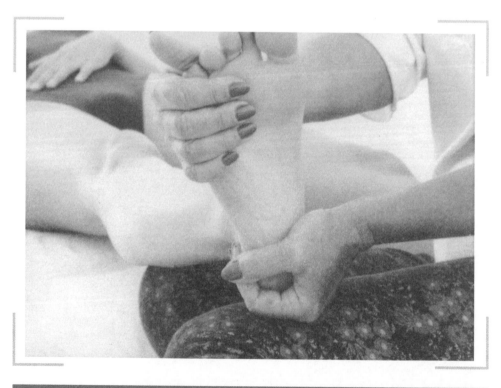

Exercise 8

The patient and the practitioner are in the same position.
The massage of the top of the foot is performed lengthwise to the toes,
one thumb on top of the other, starting from point C, where the foot and
the leg join. (See the Introduction.)

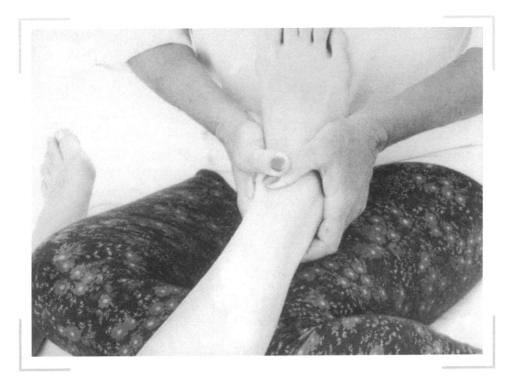

Exercise 9

The patient and the practitioner are in the same position.
The patient's leg rests on the practitioner's leg.
The practitioner massages every pair of toes separately, using turning
movements: the big toe + the baby toe, the second toe + the fourth toe,
and the middle toe by itself.
At the end of the exercise, the pads of the toes are pinched.

Comment: The massage of the big toe is particularly important because
of its connection to the spinal column.

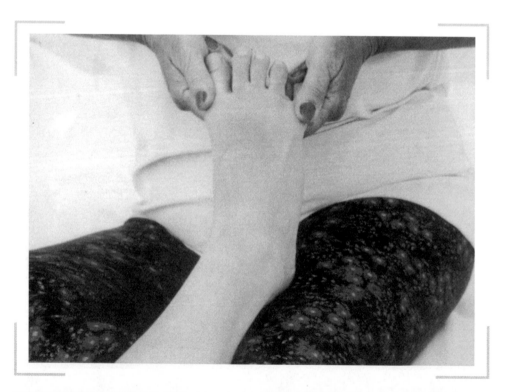

Exercise 10

The patient and the practitioner are in the same position.

The patient's foot is held between the practitioner's palms. The massage is performed by both thumbs from point C toward the toes, using turning movements, along the hollows between the bones.

At the end of the exercise, the pads of the toes are pinched.

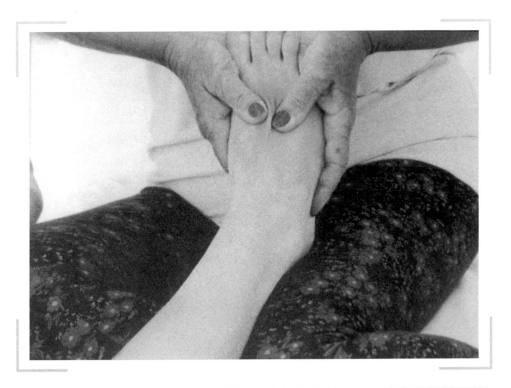

Exercise 11

The patient and the practitioner are in the same position.
With one hand, the practitioner holds the patient's foot in the region of
the muscle above the heel, and with the other, he lightly massages the
place where the toes are joined, pulling each toe separately - starting
with the big toe - and going in the direction of the baby toe.
At the end of the exercise, for relaxation: light stroking movements and
placing the foot on the floor.

Exercises 4-11 (for the sole and back of the foot)
are repeated on the other foot.

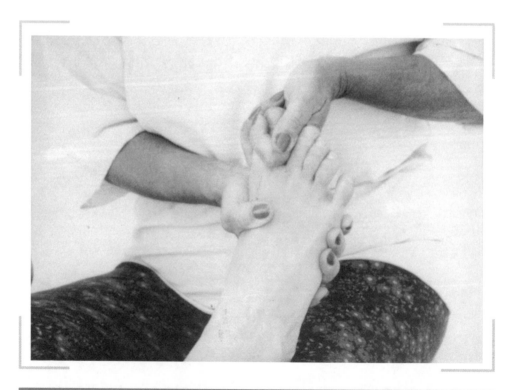

Exercise 12

The patient is in the same position.

The practitioner sits with his legs apart.

The practitioner grasps the patient's feet, crosses them, and applies pressure three times with his hands placed diagonally one on top of the other. Then he crosses the patient's feet the opposite way, and applies pressure three times, as before.

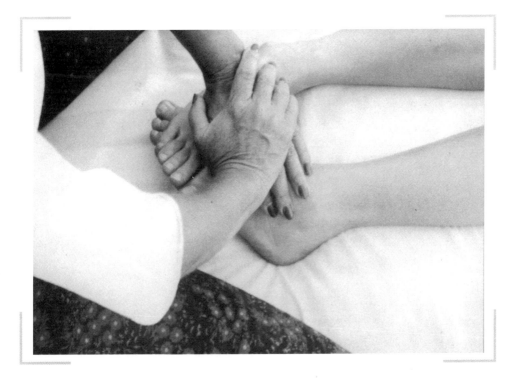

Exercise 13

The patient and the practitioner are in the same position.
The practitioner separates the patient's feet, places the soles of his feet
on the soles of the patient's feet, and applies pressure three times in the
direction of the patient's head.

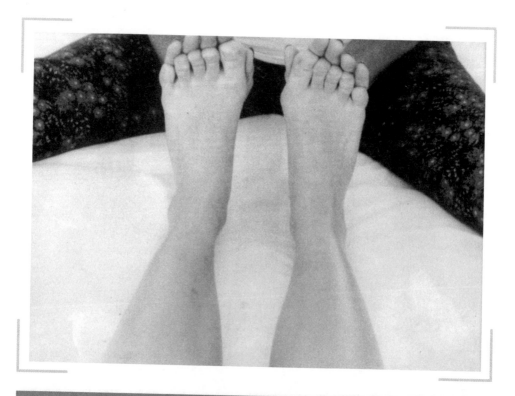

Exercise 14

The patient lies on his back.

The practitioner gets up.

One of the practitioner's knees is on the floor, while the other is slightly bent. The practitioner places both the patient's legs on his upright knee, holding them in one hand in the region above the ankle muscle, and supporting the patient's knees with his other hand.

From this position, the practitioner lifts the patient's legs up, while the hand supporting the knees applies downward pressure three times.

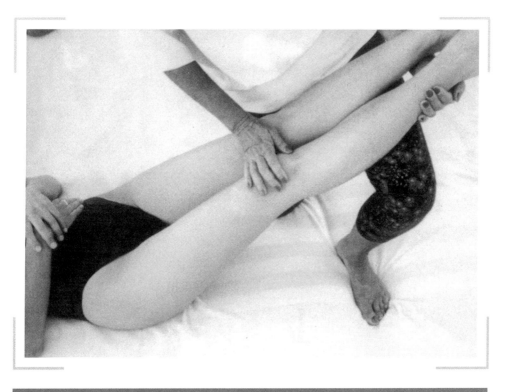

Exercise 15

The patient lies on his back.

The practitioner sits on his knees or cross-legged in the gap between the patient's legs.

The practitioner performs massage by applying pressure with his palms, starting from the sole of the patient's foot up to the groin area of the leg that is being worked on. The pressures are Walking P.P., with one hand applying pressure, the other relaxing, back and forth, several times.

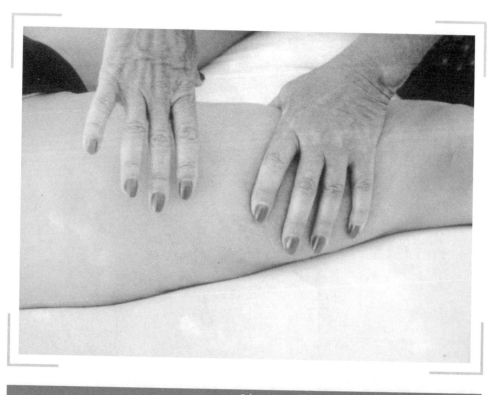

Exercise 16

The patient and the practitioner are in the same position.
The leg that is being worked on is lying on its side on the floor, with the inner part of the leg upward. The practitioner applies pressure using both thumbs (T.P.), back and forth from the ankle in the direction of the groin, along energy lines number 1 and 2.
The pressure is applied alternately: when one thumb presses, the other relaxes.

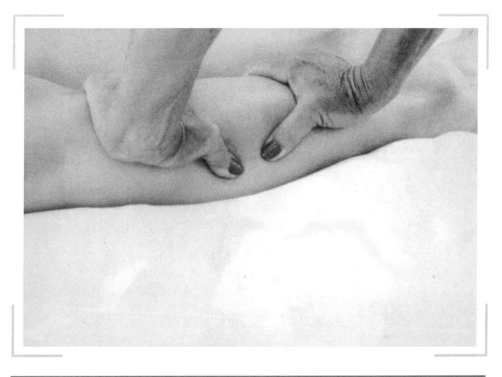

Exercise 17

The patient and the practitioner are in the same position.
The practitioner applies thumb pressure along energy line number 3 (on the inner side of the leg).

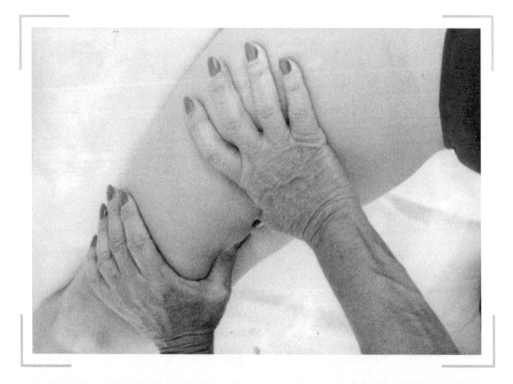

Exercise 18

The patient and the practitioner are in the same position.
The practitioner moves to the other side of the patient's leg.
The practitioner turns the patient's leg onto the outer side, upward, and
applies thumb pressure along outer energy line number 2.
This exercise can be performed without the practitioner changing sides,
but it is not comfortable.

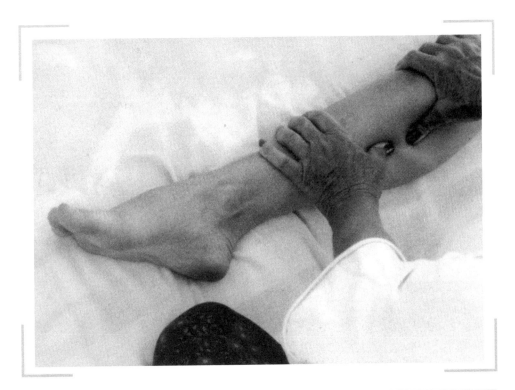

Exercise 19

The patient is in the same position.
The practitioner sits on his knees in the gap between
the patient's open legs.
Stretching: The practitioner places one hand on the patient's groin, and
holds his leg in the region above the ankle muscle with the other hand.
He stretches the leg in opposite directions.

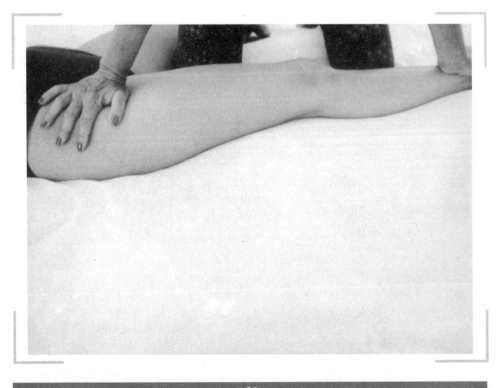

Exercise 20*

The patient lies on his back.

The practitioner stands.

Blood stopping: The practitioner places both hands, one on top of the other, on the region of the groin of the leg that is being worked on, and when he feels the flow of blood, he presses with his entire body weight for 15 to 50 seconds.

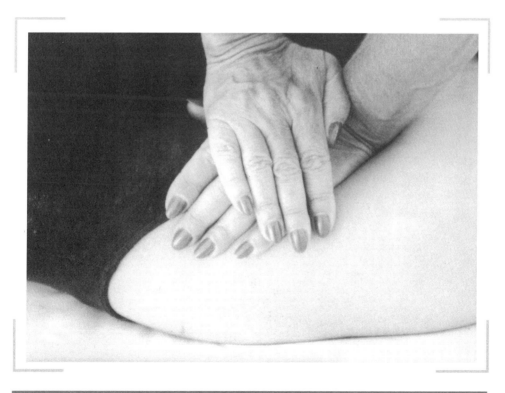

Exercise 21

The patient lies on his back.
The practitioner should be on his knees, but this depends
on how comfortable it is for him.
The exercise begins with the application of P.P. on both
of the patient's legs, from his toes to his pelvis.
The patient's leg is bent approximately at a 60-degree angle,
on the floor. The practitioner holds the knee region of the patient's
straight leg with one hand, and with the other moves upward using
Walking P.P. (the palms advancing, alternately pressing and relaxing)
on the bent leg up to the groin.

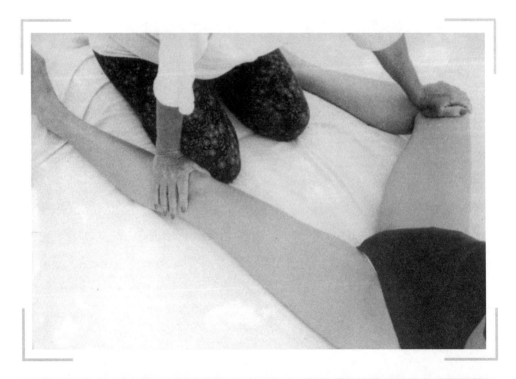

Exercise 22

The patient is in the same position.
The practitioner sits on the floor.
The practitioner widens the angle of the patient's bent leg, and holds both legs above the ankle. The practitioner places both of his feet in the area of the patient's groin, and performs "walking" movements with them. Pressure is applied with the soles of both feet, back and forth, in both directions - from the kneecap to the groin and back.
At the same time, the practitioner applies P.P. with one hand along the patient's straight leg upward - in the direction of the groin - and back again.

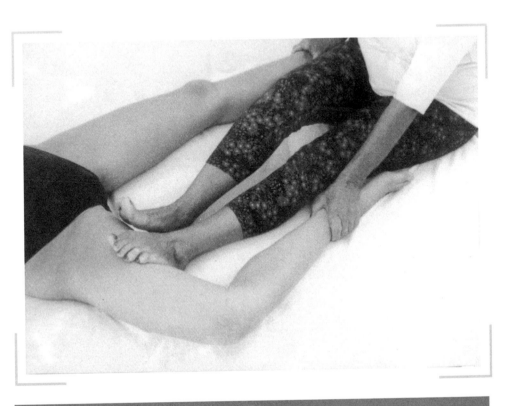

Exercise 23

The patient and the practitioner are in the same position.
The same bent leg is now placed on top of the practitioner's opposite leg (left on right), and held with one of the practitioner's hands.
The practitioner holds both of the patient's legs in the region of the muscle above the ankle.
One of the practitioner's legs remains fixed in its place - in the hollow of the patient's bent knee - and his other leg applies pressure, back and forth, to the treatment points on the inner part of the thigh, in the area between the groin and the knee.

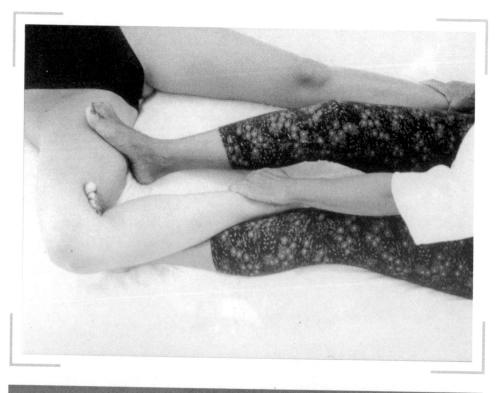

Exercise 24

The patient lies on his back.

The practitioner kneels, his buttocks resting on the soles of his feet. The leg that is being worked on is lifted, bent at a 30-degree angle, and the foot is held between the practitioner's knees, close to the floor. Both of the practitioner's hands apply alternating pressure on the area between the groin and the knee, back and forth, three times.

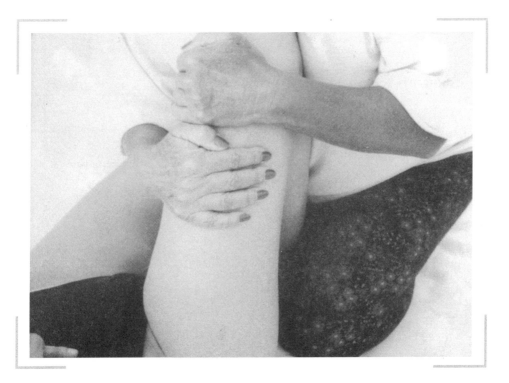

Exercise 25

The patient and the practitioner are in the same position.
The massage is performed using "squeezing" movements, with both of
the practitioner's hands pulling the leg that is being worked on, in the
area between the knee and the groin, alternately in opposite directions,
back and forth, three times.

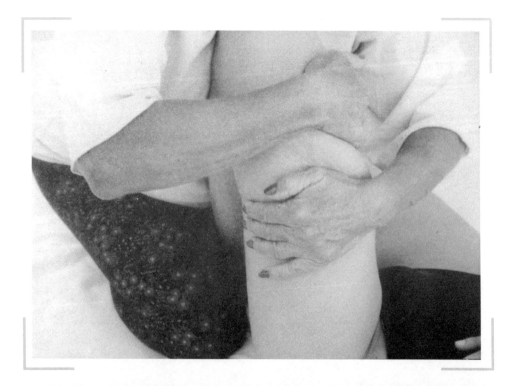

Exercise 26

The patient and the practitioner are in the same position.
The practitioner interlaces his fingers and performs massage by applying pressure with the pads of his hands, back and forth, from the knee to the groin and back.
The practitioner repeats the massage using T.P. along energy lines numbers 1 and 2 in the same area, between the knee and the groin.

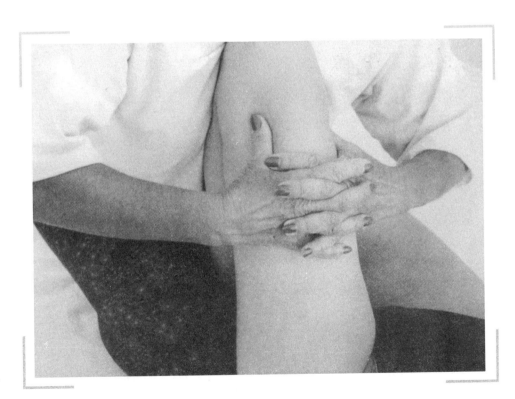

Exercise 27

The patient and the practitioner are in the same position.
The practitioner massages energy line number 3 (the central line of the back of the thigh). The massage is performed by T.P., back and forth, while the patient's thigh is held between both of the practitioner's hands. During the next part of the exercise, pressure is applied alternately by the palms, back and forth in a "walking" movement, and then in a "twisting" movement.

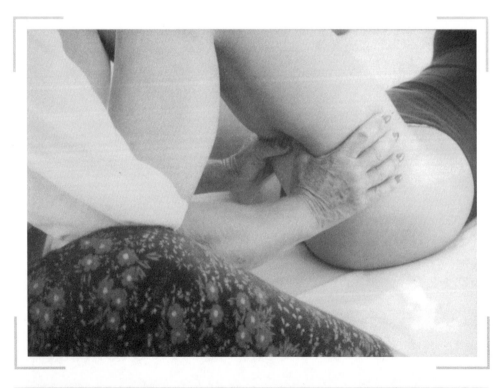

Exercise 28

The patient is in the same position.
The practitioner is seated with legs apart.
The foot that is being worked on is supported by the practitioner's thigh.
The massage is performed on the calf.
The practitioner interlaces his fingers and massages the patient's calf,
back and forth, from the area of the kneecap in the direction of the ankle,
using the pads of his hands. Afterward, he applies T.P. along
the energy lines.
At the end of the exercise, he applies Walking P.P. back and forth
along the calf.

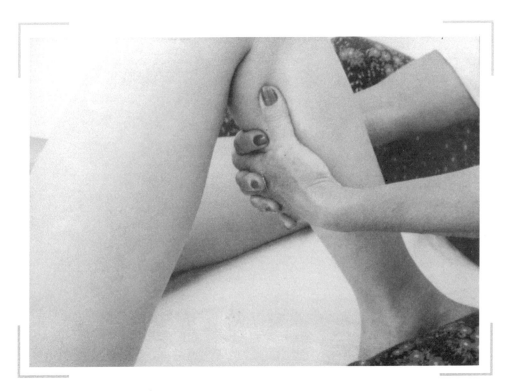

Exercise 29

The patient lies on his back.

The practitioner sits on his knees.

With one knee, the practitioner supports the patient's straight leg in the area of the knee, and he inserts his other knee into the hollow of the patient's other kneecap.

With one hand, the practitioner holds the patient's bent knee, and with his other hand, he applies pressure back and forth along the thigh, from the groin to the knee.

The aim of the exercise is for the practitioner to use his body to push the patient's bent leg three times in the direction of his head.

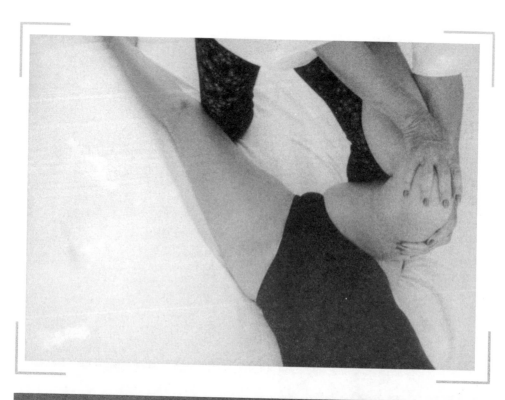

Exercise 30

The patient is in the same position.

The practitioner sits on the floor.

The angle of the leg that is being worked on is increased to 90 degrees.

The practitioner holds the leg that is being worked on in both hands, one hand holding the area of the ankle, and the other holding the calf.

The practitioner places one of his feet on the back part of the patient's thigh (of the bent leg). His other foot performs "walking" movements back and forth along the back part of the patient's thigh. Counter pressure is applied to the leg that is being worked on - the practitioner uses his hands to pull it toward his body, and his legs to push it away from his body (stretching).

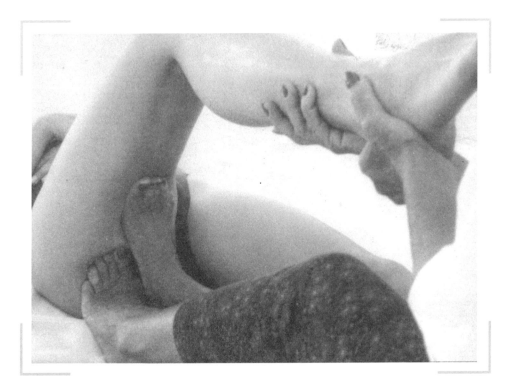

Exercise 31

The patient and the practitioner are in the same position.
The practitioner holds the back of the leg that is being worked on in one
hand, and the calf - in the region of the ankle - in the other.
One of the practitioner's legs is close to the leg that is being worked on,
in the inner region of the thigh, and his other leg is beneath
the patient's straight leg.
The practitioner pulls the leg that is being worked on toward him, while
leaning his body backward in the direction of the floor.
Pressure is applied by means of moving the practitioner's foot from
point to point, relaxing between points.

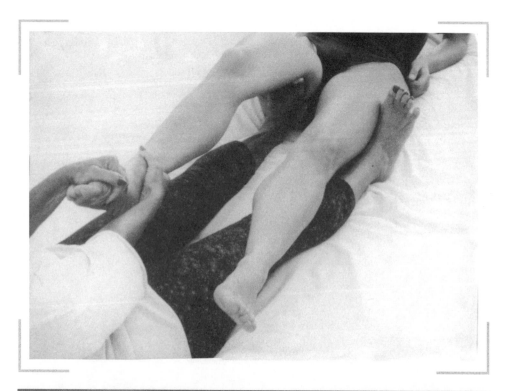

Exercise 32

The patient is in the same position.

The practitioner sits on his knees.

The patient's leg is bent downward, as close as possible to the floor, with the outer angle between the calf and the thigh being 30 degrees. His knee is supported by the practitioner's knees.

Using his hands, the practitioner massages the patient's bent leg alternately, back and forth, performing "walking" movements from the knee to the pelvis and back.

The exercise can also be performed when the patient's knee is not on the floor, but rather between the practitioner's knees. Afterward, the practitioner performs "chopping" massage - both palms together applying rapid "hammer blows" back and forth.

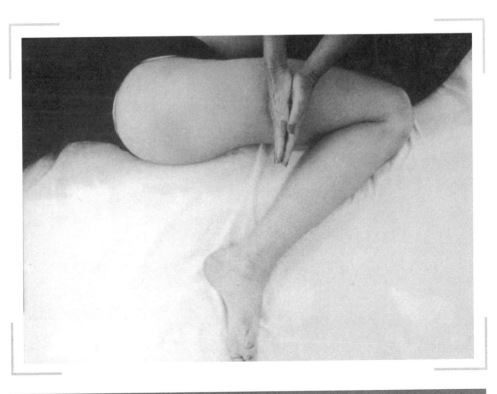

Exercise 33

The patient is in the same position.
The practitioner moves to the patient's side, with one knee on the floor, and his other leg bent at a 90-degree angle.
The practitioner holds the area of the patient's ankle in one hand, while the other holds the thigh in the groin area. This leg is raised to a 30-degree angle, and is supported on the practitioner's knee. The raised foot touches the practitioner's forearm. The practitioner performs two movements simultaneously:
With one hand, he pulls the leg that is being held in the region of the ankle outward.
With the other hand, he pulls the groin area in the opposite direction.
(The exercise is stretching the leg.)
At the end of the exercise, the practitioner places the patient's raised leg gently on the floor, after shaking it lightly.

Exercises 14-33 are repeated on the other leg.

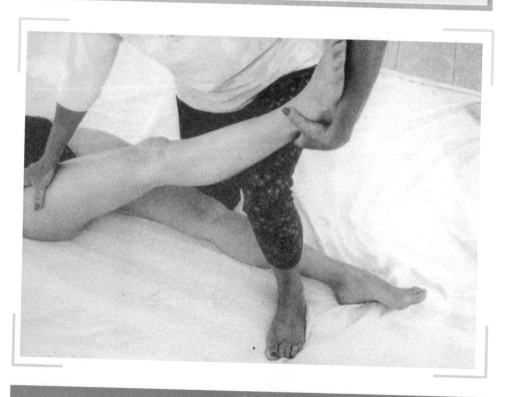

Exercise 34

The patient lies on his back.

The practitioner stands opposite him.

The practitioner's left leg supports the patient's body in the region of the waist. The practitioner lifts the patient's legs to a 90-degree angle, leaning both the patient's legs to the left, while holding them above the region of the ankle. With his right hand, the practitioner holds the patient's feet, and he places his left hand on the back of the patient's feet, above the ankle area.

At this stage, the practitioner applies pressure with his entire body to the patient's legs, which are close together, and leans them in the direction of the patient's head. (The patient ostensibly moves his legs over his head.)

The exercise is repeated twice more.

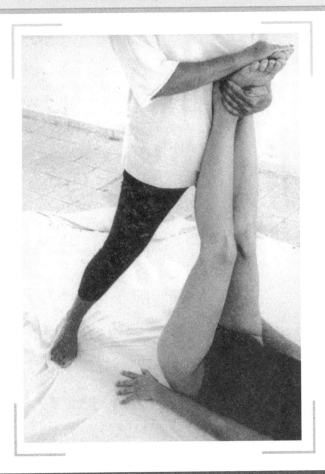

Exercise 35

The patient lies on his back.
The practitioner stands.
The patient's left leg is raised at a 90-degree angle, touching the practitioner's right leg, and held in the region above the ankle by both the practitioner's hands. The patient's right leg is bent, with his right foot between the area of his left knee and the practitioner's right leg. The practitioner's left leg is in front of the patient's bent leg, pushing it toward himself, while his foot supports the patient's waist.
In this position, the practitioner moves his body forward and backward three times.

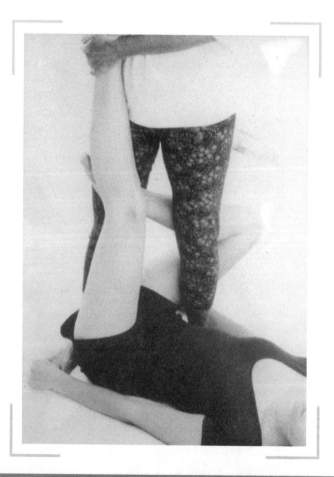

Exercise 36

The patient and the practitioner are in the same position.
The practitioner holds the patient's leg upright in his left hand, above the ankle. He uses his right forearm to apply pressure to the patient's lifted foot, back and forth in a sliding movement. This exercise must be performed twice, back and forth.

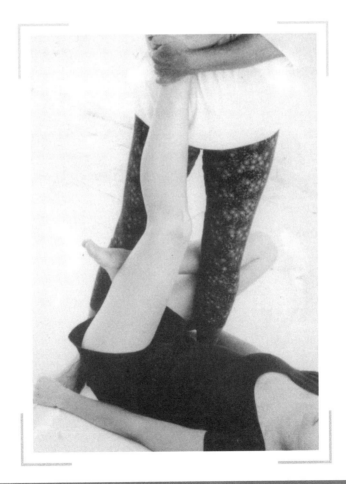

Exercise 37

The patient and the practitioner are in the same position.
The practitioner applies pressure with his elbow to the six treatment points on the patient's foot (see the diagram of the foot in the Introduction), while his other hand holds the leg that is being worked on above the ankle.
Afterward, the practitioner performs sliding movements with his forearms, backward and forward.
At the end, he administers punches to the foot that is being worked on, back and forth, twice.

Comment: Care must be taken on the bones.

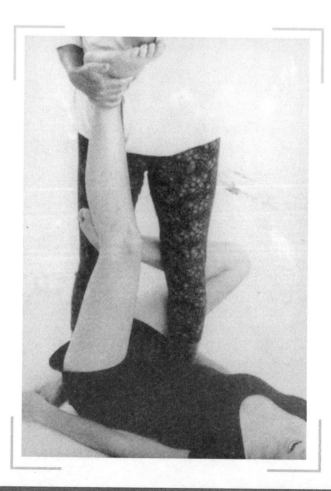

Exercise 38

The patient and the practitioner are in the same position.
The practitioner moves the patient's raised leg onto his right shoulder,
his right hand holding the leg by the knee.
In his other hand, the practitioner holds the bent leg in the knee area,
using it to apply pressure to the patient's knee toward the floor, and
trying to move it away from his supporting leg.
With his other hand and leg, the practitioner applies counter pressure.
At the end of the exercise, the patient's legs are close together and lying
on the floor.

Exercises 35-38 are repeated on the other leg.

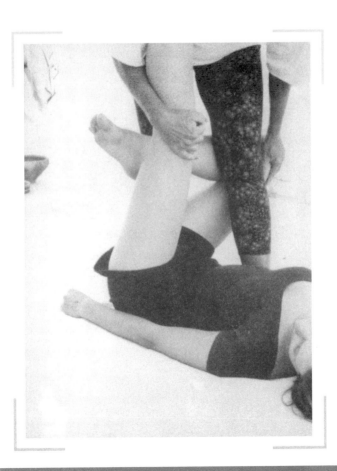

Exercise 39*

The patient lies on his back.
The practitioner stands.
The practitioner lifts and bends the patient's legs, which are close together, while holding the upper surface of the patient's feet. At this stage, the practitioner places his knees on the patient's inner thighs, while pushing and pulling his feet.

* This pressure is applied along the three treatment points of the inner thigh, from the knees toward the pelvis.

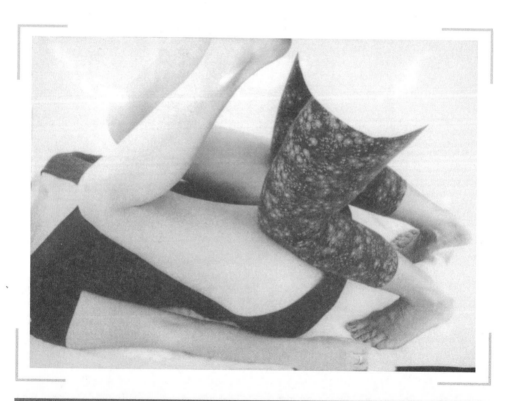

Exercise 40

The patient lies on his back.
The practitioner stands.
The patient's feet are on the practitioner's chest.
The practitioner's legs are wide apart, and support the patient's body
in the area of his waist.
The practitioner's hands hold the patient's hands in the area
of the forearms.
The practitioner pulls the patient's arm upward, and lifts him three times,
each time higher than the last.

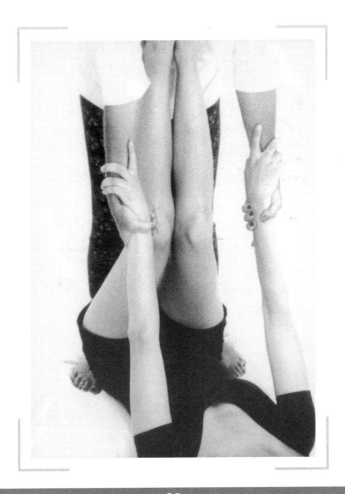

Exercise 41

The patient and the practitioner are in the same position.
The patient crosses his legs and places them on the practitioner's shins.
The patient's hands hold the practitioner's forearms, and the practitioner
pulls him upward three times, as high as possible.

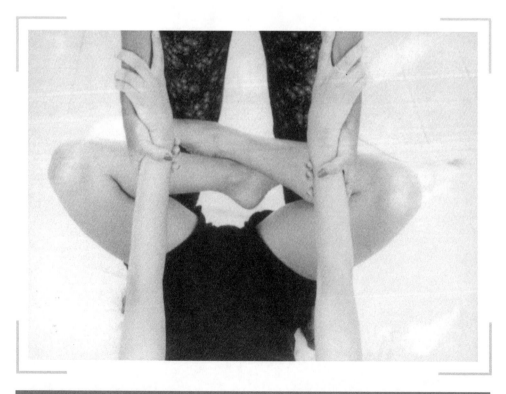

Exercise 42

The patient and the practitioner are in the same position.
The practitioner pulls the patient to himself three times, and on the third
time he seats the patient in a cross-legged position,
his palms on the floor.

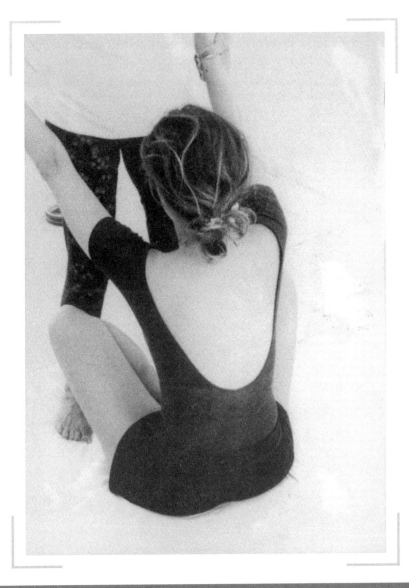

Massaging Nack and Shoulders (Ex. 43-50)

Exercise 43

The patient sits cross-legged.
The practitioner stands behind him.
The practitioner uses both hands simultaneously to massages the patient's shoulders, applying the weight of his entire body.
P.P. is applied back and forth from the neck to the shoulders and back, several times.

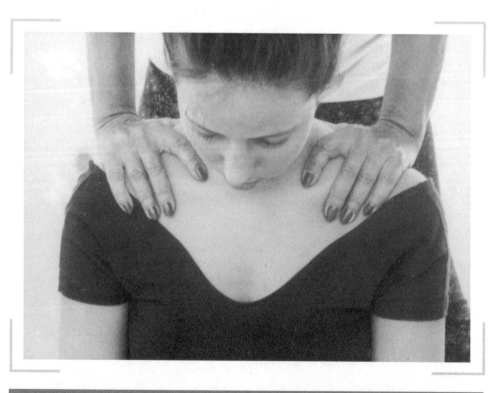

Exercise 44

The patient and the practitioner are in the same position.
The massage is performed by T.P. on the three treatment points, from
the neck to the shoulders, back and forth. (See the diagram
of the treatment points.)
The practitioner's fingers on both hands hold on to the front
of the patient's shoulders.
At the end of the exercise, a rotate massage by thumb pressure
is performed.

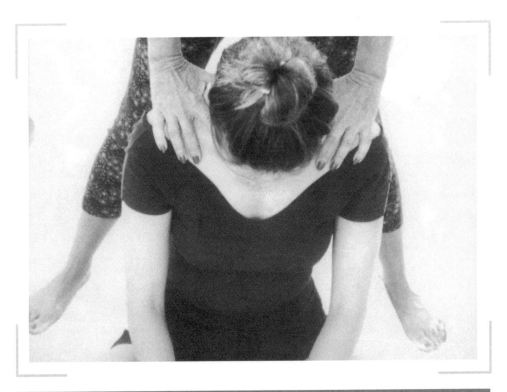

Exercise 45

The patient and the practitioner are in the same position.
The massage is performed by the thumbs, which apply pressure to the front side of the shoulders in turning movements, while the practitioner's hands hold on to the back of the shoulders.

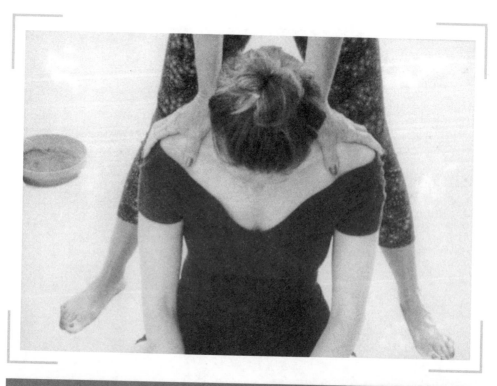

Exercise 46

The patient and the practitioner are in the same position.
The practitioner performs a "chopping" exercise on the patient's
shoulders, from the neck along the shoulder, back and forth, and then
along the back, except in the region of the spine.
The exercise ends with both the practitioner's hands stroking the
patient's shoulders and back.

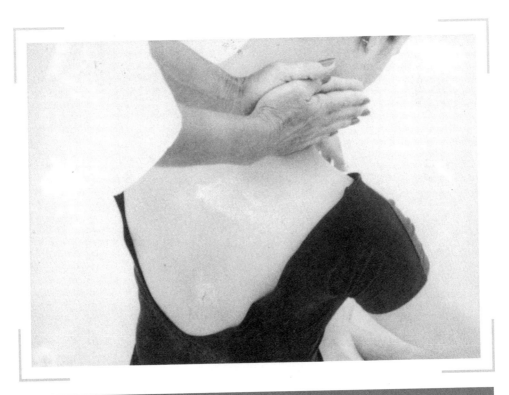

Exercise 47

The patient sits cross-legged, his head bowed.
The practitioner is behind him, one knee on the floor, and the other lifted and supporting the patient's back. His forearms rest on the patient's shoulders and slide back and forth, applying all the strength of his body to the patient's body.

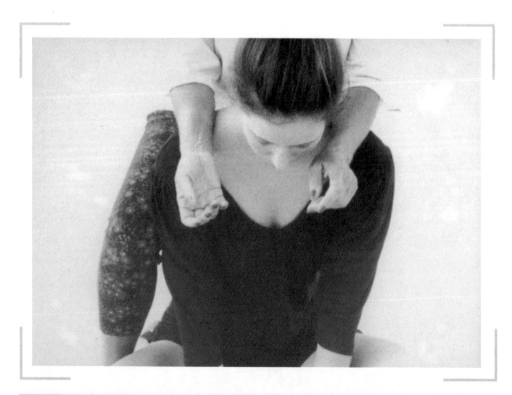

Exercise 48*

The patient and the practitioner are in the same position.
The practitioner interlaces his fingers, and uses them to bend the patient's head to one side, applying the pressure with his body on the shoulder by means of his elbow.
The exercise is performed on several points along the shoulder, with great caution, applying light pressure.
The exercise is repeated on the other shoulder.

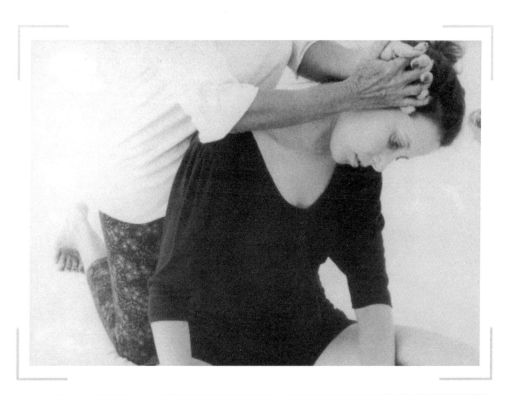

Exercise 49

The patient and the practitioner are in the same position.
The practitioner bends one of the patient's arms backward, grasping his
elbow in one hand, and holding his upper arm against his body.
While one of the practitioner's hands holds the elbow, the other
massages the upper arm, back and forth, several times.

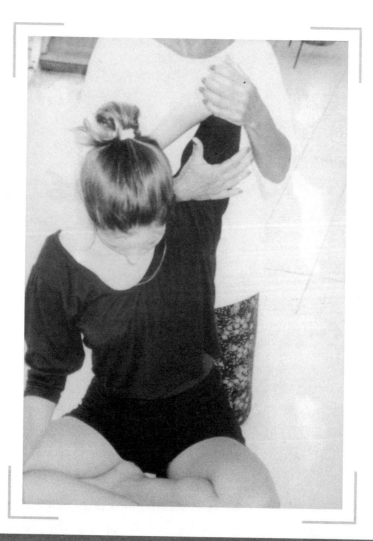

Exercise 50*

The patient is in the same position.
The practitioner sits behind the patient, his knees on the floor.
One of the practitioner's knees touches the patient's lower back. With one hand, he bends the patient's arm backward, supporting the patient's shoulder with his elbow, and holding the patient's fingers. With the other hand, the practitioner holds the patient's elbow.
The massage is performed by means of the elbow moving along the patient's shoulder, all the while pulling the patient's arm backward.
At the end of the exercise, "shaking" is performed
on the patient's upper arm.

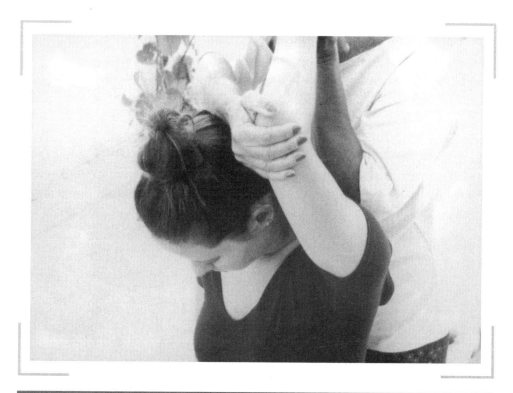

Abdominal Massage (Ex. 51-54)

This massage must be performed on an empty stomach
(at least three hours after a meal).
The direction of the rotate massage depends on the purpose of the
treatment. If constipation is being treated, the rotate massage goes from
left to right - in a clockwise direction. If diarrhea is being treated, the
rotate massage goes from right to left, in an anti-clockwise direction.
(Regulating the digestive system is a clockwise movement, which is why
a massage for treating constipation must be performed in a clockwise
direction, and for treating diarrhea must be performed in an
anti-clockwise direction.)

Exercise 51

The patient lies on his back.
(Women - with their legs bent, knees upward. Men - with their legs
straight, resting on the floor.)
The practitioner moves to the patient's side. The treatment begins with a
massage of the legs (exercises 1-3). On the abdomen, there are six
massage treatment points (see the diagram of the abdomen in the
Introduction). The practitioner applies pressure with the pads of his
palms, one on top of the other, to point number 1.
The massage along the six points goes in a circular/turning direction.

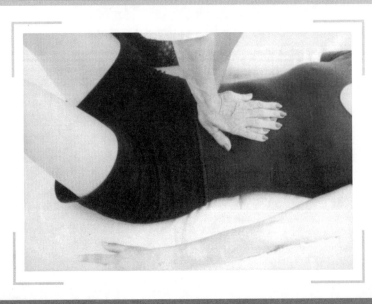

Exercise 52

The patient and the practitioner are in the same position.
The massage is performed with the palms placed one on top of the other
diagonally. Each point must be massaged separately, using a circular/
turning movement.
Each point is massaged for five seconds.

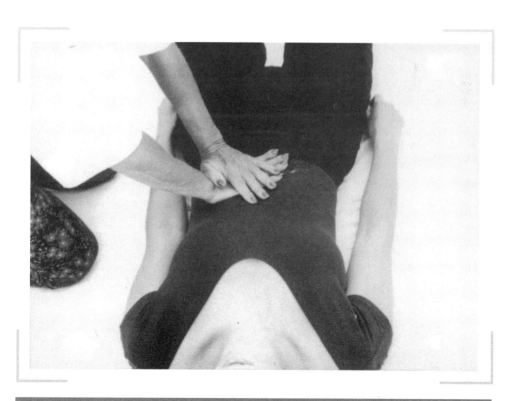

Exercise 53

The patient and the practitioner are in the same position.
The massage is performed on the six treatment points, using both thumbs, while the palms support the abdomen at the same time, on every pair of points. Pressure is applied to each point for five seconds. After applying pressure, the practitioner performs rotation massage in the region of the point.

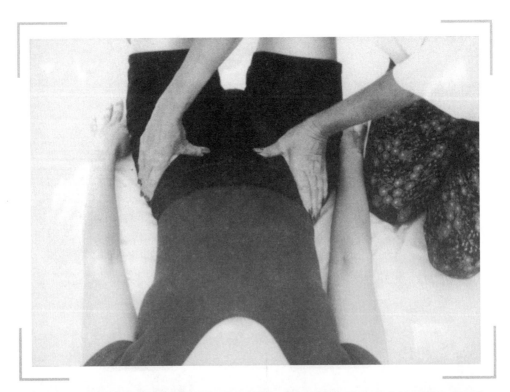

Exercise 54

The patient and the practitioner are in the same position.
The massage is a repetition of applying pressure by the thumbs, followed
by rotation movements, while the practitioner's palms hold the patient's
body near the waist, and move upward.
The pressures are applied from the side toward the center of the body.

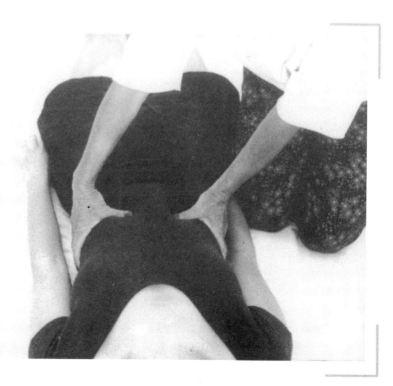

Massage of the Chest and the Upper Arms (Ex. 55-63)

Exercise 55

The patient lies on his back.
The practitioner kneels beside him.
The patient's legs are straight and closed.
The practitioner massages using three fingers - the forefinger, the middle finger, and the fourth finger - along the chest cavity up to the neck.
The massage consists of pressures and rotation movements.

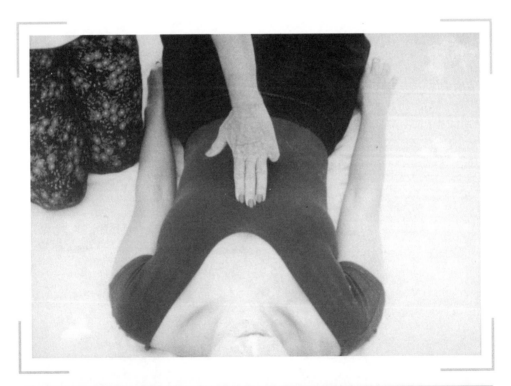

Exercise 56

The patient lies on his back.
The practitioner sits on his knees, leaning over the patient's body.
The practitioner's palms grasp the back of the patient's shoulder-blades
and massage them gently, back and forth, using P.P.

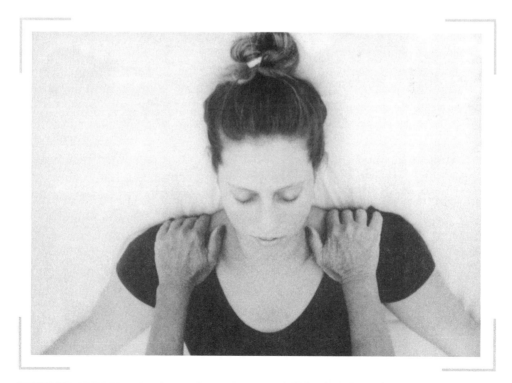

Exercise 57

The patient and the practitioner are in the same position.
The massage is performed by the thumbs, simultaneously on both
shoulders, back and forth, using T.P.

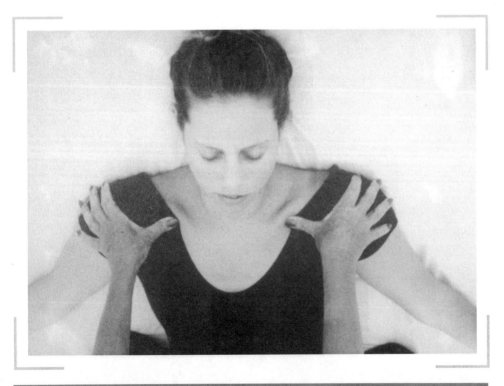

Exercise 58

The patient and the practitioner are in the same position.
The massage starts with P.P. on the shoulders, back and forth.
Then the practitioner's palms grasp the patient's shoulders firmly, and
the practitioner lifts the patient's body, while applying pressure to the
muscles of the shoulder-blades, three times, lifting higher each time.

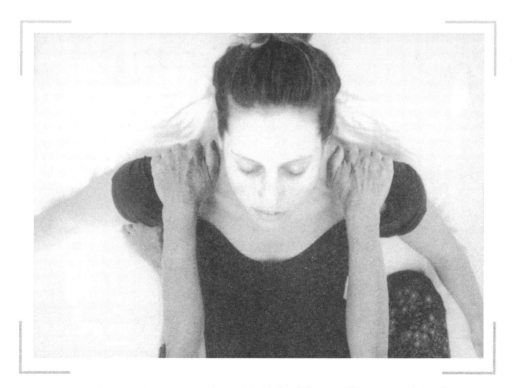

Exercise 59

The patient lies on his back.
The practitioner stands, bending over the patient.
The practitioner's palms hold the patient's body in the region of the lower back. His fingers apply pressure to the muscles. The practitioner lifts the patient's body three times. The patient's head and legs rest on the floor.

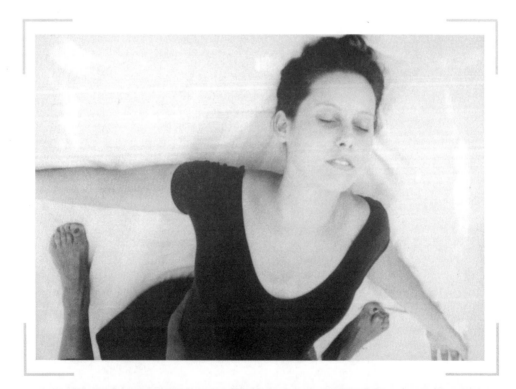

Exercise 60

The patient lies on his back, with one arm resting on the floor, extended at right angles to his body.
The practitioner sits on his knees.
(Men - start with the right arm. Women - start with the left arm.)
The practitioner sits close to the extended arm and massages it from the wrist up to the armpit, using walking P.P.

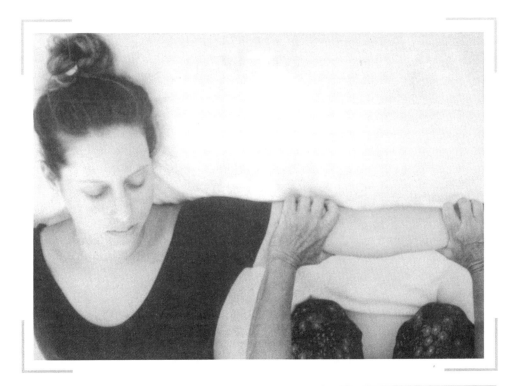

Exercise 61

The patient and the practitioner are in the same position.
The massage is performed by T.P., alternately, back and forth along the
two energy lines of the inner arm.
The next part of the massage is performed with walking P.P.

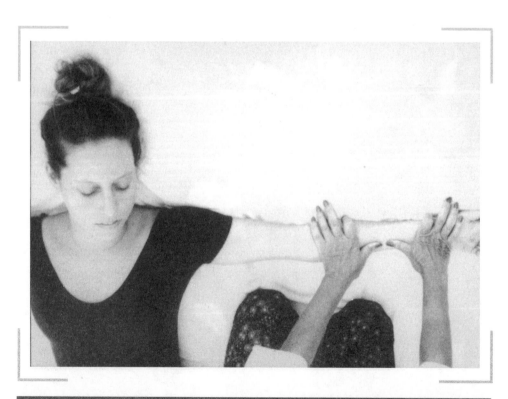

Exercise 62

The patient and the practitioner are in the same position.
In one hand, the practitioner holds the patient's extended arm in the
region of the armpit, while his other hand holds the wrist. He pulls in
opposite directions once - stretching.

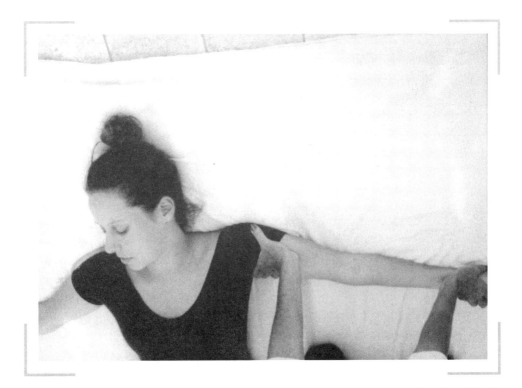

Exercise 63

The patient and the practitioner are in the same position.
Blood stopping by applying pressure to the armpit, using both palms,
one on top of the other, for 15-30 seconds, once.

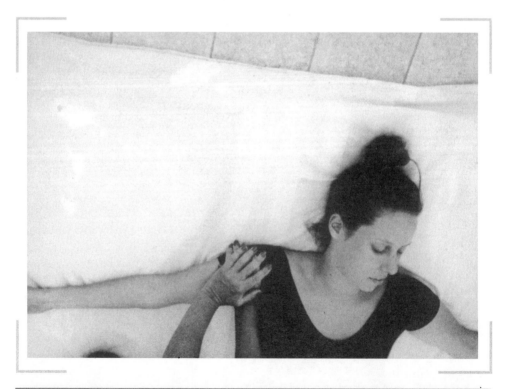

The Massage of the Palm (Ex. 64-74)

Exercise 64

The patient lies on his back.
The practitioner sits cross-legged, or in another comfortable position.
The patient's arm rests on a pillow, or on the practitioner's knees. The massage of the palm starts with both of the practitioner's thumbs, one on top of the other, applying gentle pressure to the point in the middle of the palm, and then in the direction of the fingers. Pressure is applied to each point for five seconds, three times per point. The treatment ends with rotation massage (see the diagram of the palm in the Introduction).

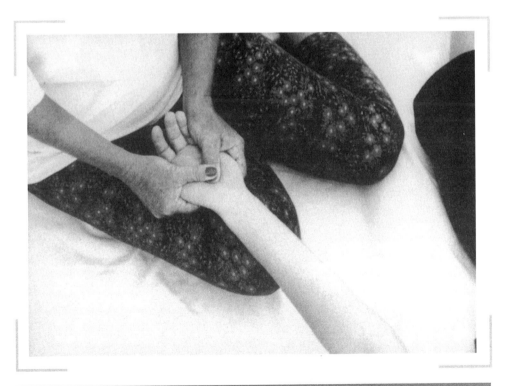

Exercise 65

The patient and the practitioner are in the same position.
The practitioner interlaces his fingers with the patient's fingers and massages the patient's palm, using rotation movements. The massage moves from the wrist toward the fingers. Afterward, the practitioner releases the patient's fingers, grasps his pinkie and thumb in both hands, and massages by with rotation movements, from the base of the fingers to their tips, several times.
Finally, using both hands, the whole palm is massaged, and when the pads of the fingers are reached, they are massaged well and pinched.

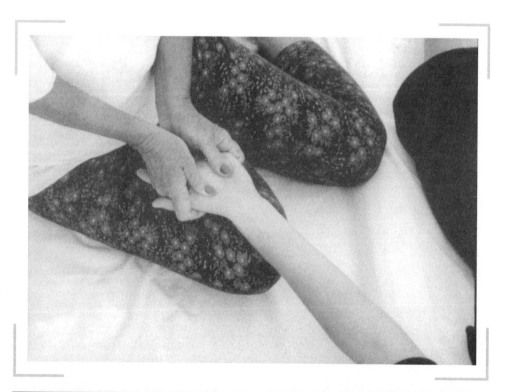

Exercise 66

The patient and the practitioner are in the same position.
The massage is performed on the upper surface of the patient's hand.
The practitioner performs rotation movements with his thumbs along the
hollows between the bones of the fingers, from the wrist to the fingers,
beginning at the join of the upper surface of the hand (point A). The
practitioner's thumbs are placed one on top of the other, and apply
pressure to this point for about five seconds, and continue up to the
fingertips with rotation movements.

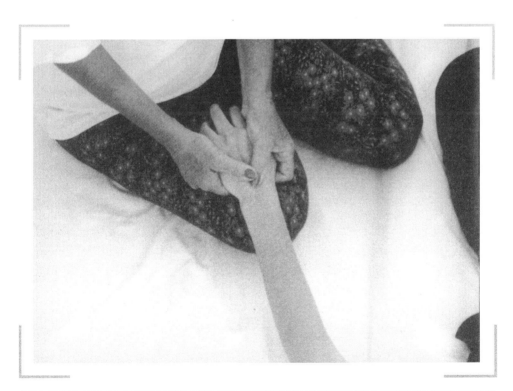

Exercise 67

The patient and the practitioner are in the same position.
The massage begins at point A by applying T.P. and rotation
on each pair of fingers for five seconds.

The order of the massage:
Thumb and pinkie.
Forefinger and fourth finger.
Middle finger.

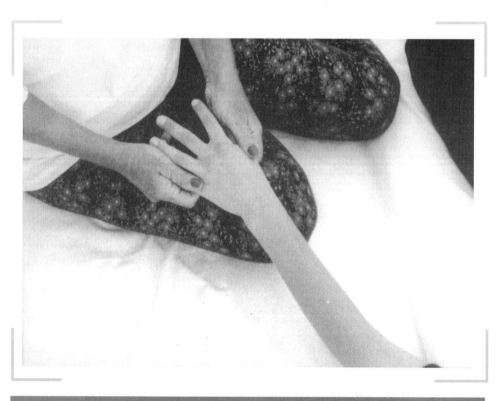

Exercise 68

The patient and the practitioner are in the same position.
The practitioner holds the patient's forearm in his left hand, and
interlaces the fingers of his right hand with the fingers of the patient's
left hand. The practitioner grasps the patient's hand firmly and rotates it
left and right three times.

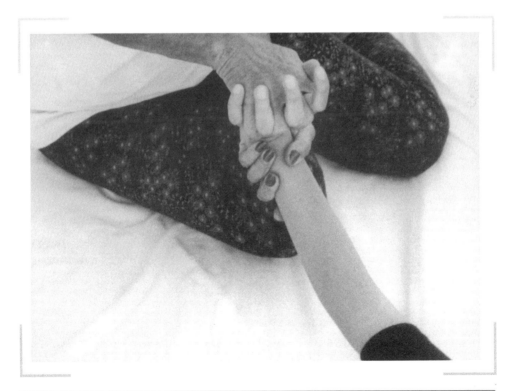

Exercise 69

The patient and the practitioner are in the same position.
The practitioner uses his fingers to press the patient's hand in the direction of the patient's head three times, and in the opposite direction - toward the practitioner - three times.
The exercise ends by rotating the hand three times in each direction.

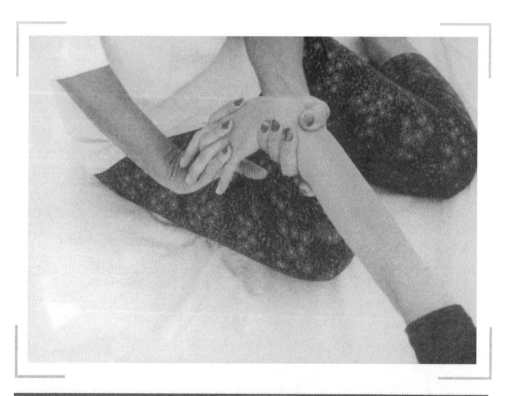

Exercise 70

The patient and the practitioner are in the same position.
The practitioner massages each of the patient's fingers with one hand,
from point A to the fingertip, using rotation movements, along the bones
of the upper surface of the hand.
After the massage of each finger, the practitioner uses his other hand to
stretch the patient's finger between his fingers, until a "cracking"
sound is heard.

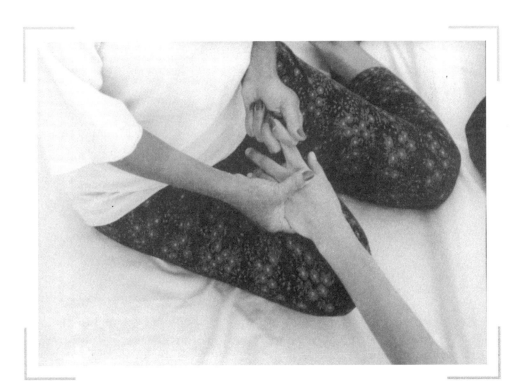

Exercise 71

The patient and the practitioner are in the same position.
One of the patient's arms rests at the side of his body, while his other arm is bent backward, the upper arm touching his head, the elbow pointing upward, and the palm on the floor.
The practitioner holds the patient's upright elbow in one hand, and uses his other hand to massage the upper arm by P.P.
Then the practitioner performs a massage using "chopping" and "shaking" movements.

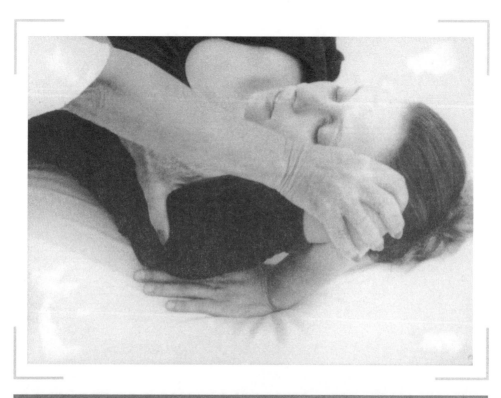

Exercise 72

The patient lies on his back. The arm that is being worked on is close to his body, its outer side upward.

The practitioner kneels at the patient's side.

The practitioner performs a massage by P.P., along the whole arm, back and forth.

(The massage can be repeated several times.)

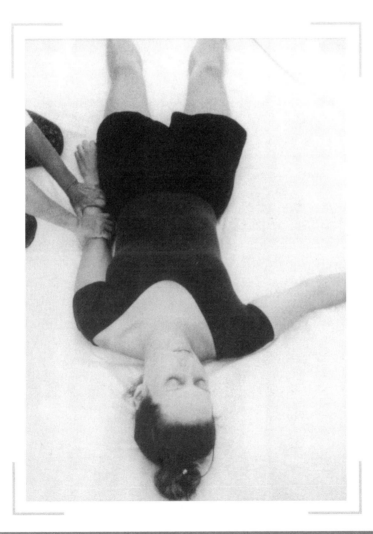

Exercise 73

The patient and the practitioner are in the same position.
The practitioner uses T.P. back and forth along the second outer energy
line to massage the arm that is being worked on.

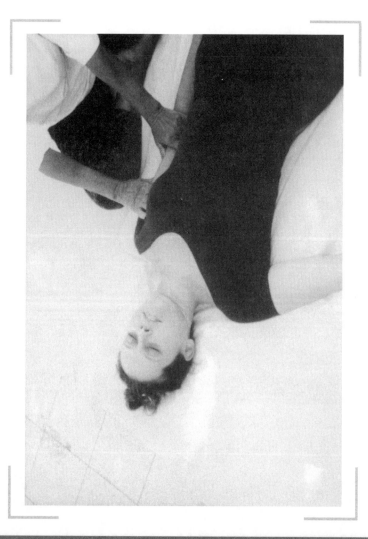

Exercise 74

The patient and the practitioner are in the same position.
The practitioner uses "squeezing" movements back and forth, and finishes with P.P.

Exercises 60-74 are repeated on the other arm.

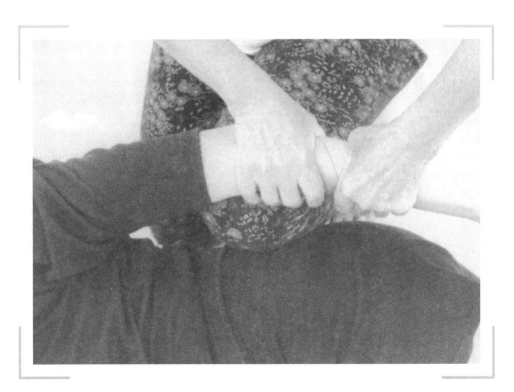

Massage Exercises Lying on Either Side (Ex. 75-128)

Exercise 75

The patient lies on his side, his head resting on his arm. The patient's opposite leg is bent, with the knee upward.
(Women - the massage begins on the left leg. Men - on the right leg.)
The practitioner kneels next to the straight leg, and uses walking P.P. back and forth from the toes toward the groin.
This exercise must be repeated several times.

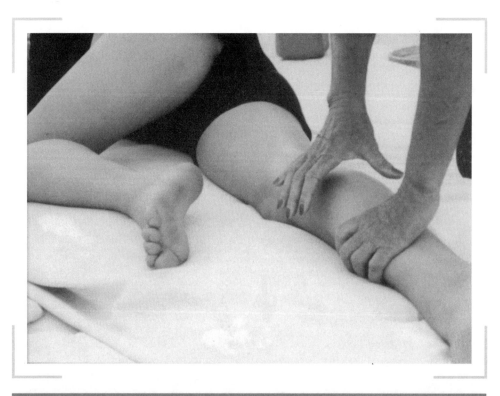

Exercise 76

The patient and the practitioner are in the same position.
T.P. is applied along the energy lines, ending with P.P.

Comment: Pressure is not applied to the kneecap - just
rotation movements.

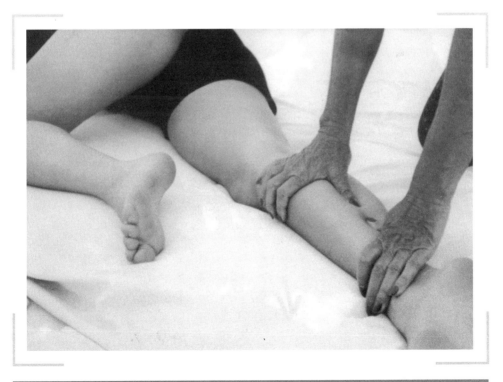

Exercise 77

The patient and the practitioner are in the same position.
The practitioner holds the patient's leg at two points: one hand in the groin region, and the other on the muscle above the ankle.
From this position, the practitioner stretches the leg by pulling it in opposite directions.

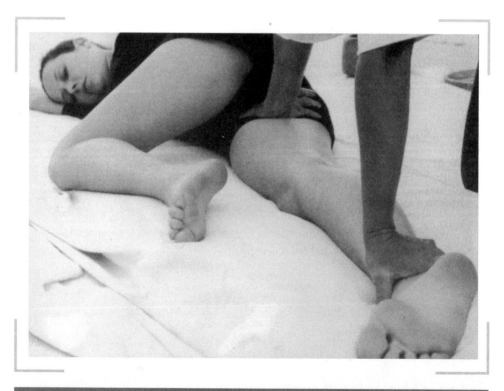

Exercise 78

The patient and the practitioner are in the same position.
The practitioner places his hands one on top of the other, diagonally, lays them on the groin and pushes with his entire body weight for 15 to 50 seconds, in order to stop the flow of blood (as in Exercise 20).
Finally, the practitioner applies P.P., back and forth, to the leg that is being worked on.

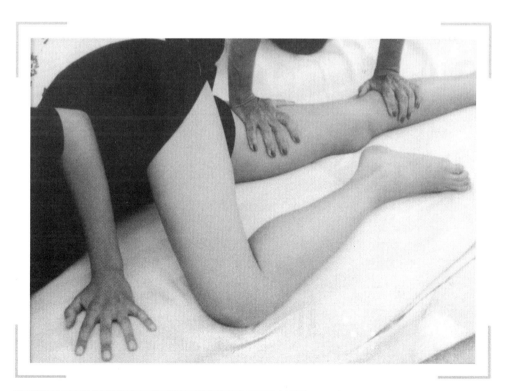

Exercise 79

The patient and the practitioner are in the same position.
The massage is performed on the bent leg, and begins with P.P., back and forth, three times.
The direction of the massage is from the knee to the ankle with one hand, and from the knee to the groin with the other.

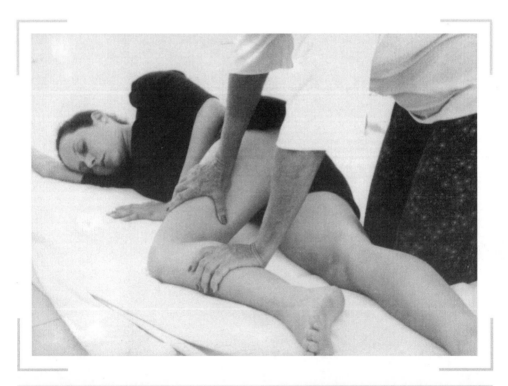

Exercise 80

The patient and the practitioner are in the same position.
The massage is performed by T.P., back and forth, along the outside
energy lines number 2 and 3, from the ankle to the groin and back.

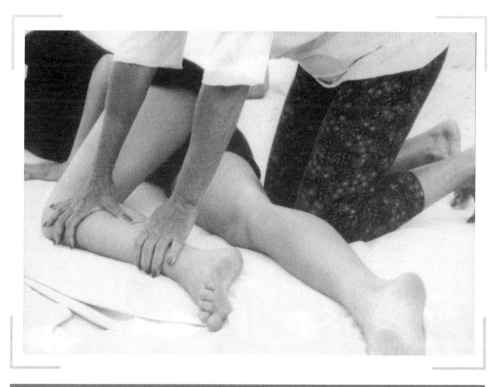

Exercise 81

The patient and the practitioner are in the same position.
The practitioner holds the patient's foot in the region above the toes in
one hand, and in the other, he holds the patient's knee, and pulls in
opposite directions (calf stretching).

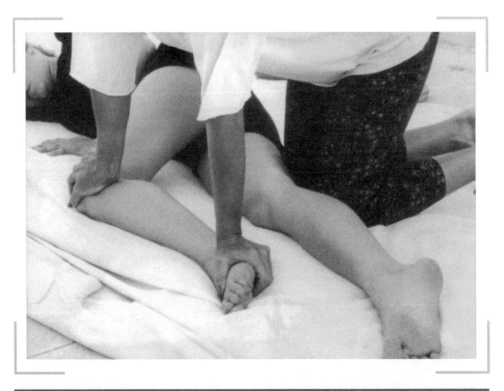

Exercise 82

The patient and the practitioner are in the same position.
The practitioner holds the patient's bent leg in the region of the knee in one hand, and in the other, he holds the region of the pelvis, and pulls the thigh in opposite directions (thigh stretching).

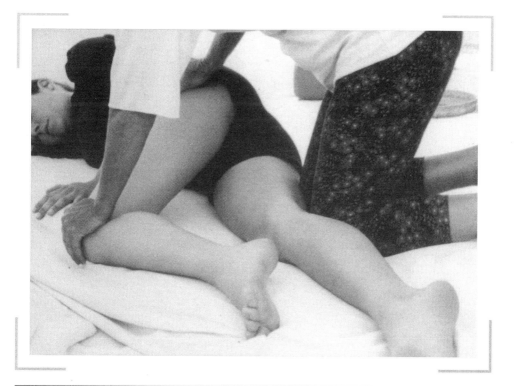

Exercise 83

The patient is in the same position.
The practitioner sits in the space between the patient's legs.
The practitioner pushes the patient's bent knee onto the floor, while
holding both the patient's legs in his two hands above the ankle.
The practitioner applies pressure with both feet in a "walking"
movement to the back of the patient's thigh,
back and forth, alternately.

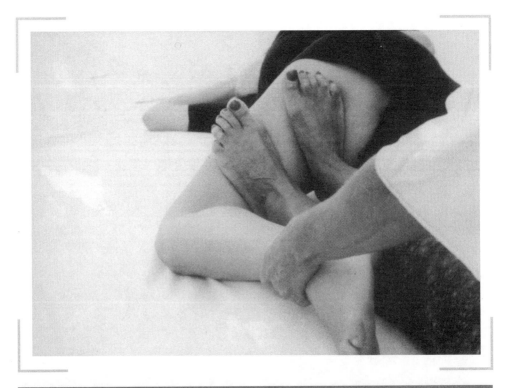

Exercice 84

The patient and the practitioner are in the same position.
The practitioner inserts his foot into the angle of the patient's bent knee,
holding the ankle of the leg that is being worked on in his hand.
The practitioner uses his other foot to apply pressure to the three
treatment points on the back of the thigh, back and forth.

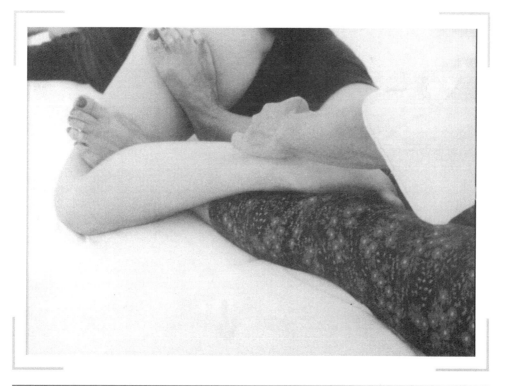

Exercise 85

The patient and the practitioner are in the same position.
The practitioner lifts the patient's bent leg, thigh upward, and inserts
both feet behind the patient's knee. The practitioner holds the outer side
of the patient's thigh in his hands, and applies walking P.P., while pulling
the thigh toward him.

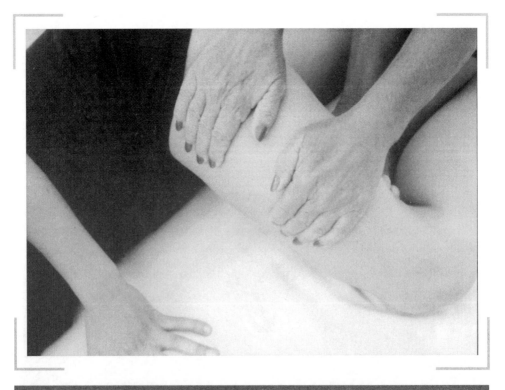

Exercise 86

The patient and the practitioner are in the same position.
The massage is performed with the fists along the thigh, back and forth,
alternately, from the area of the groin to the knee.

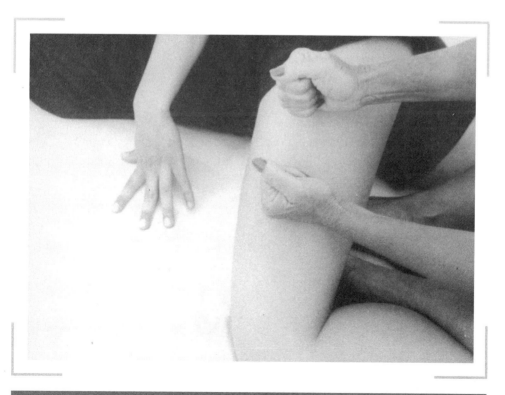

Exercise 87

The patient lies on his side.
The practitioner sits on his knees at the patient's side.
The practitioner crosses his hands and performs circle massage above
the thigh bone, several times in each direction.

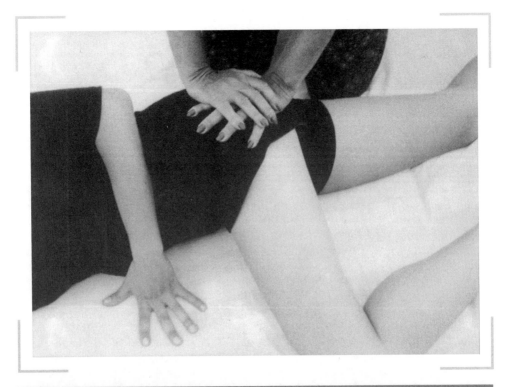

Exercise 88*

The patient and the practitioner are in the same position.
The practitioner places one thumb on top of the other and applies
pressure to points 2 and 3 (see the diagram of treatment points in the
Introduction) for about five seconds each.
Then he performs turning movements with both thumbs.
Afterward, the practitioner massages along the outer energy lines of the
leg, back and forth, using P.P., T.P., and finally relaxation by P.P.
The exercise ends with stretching.

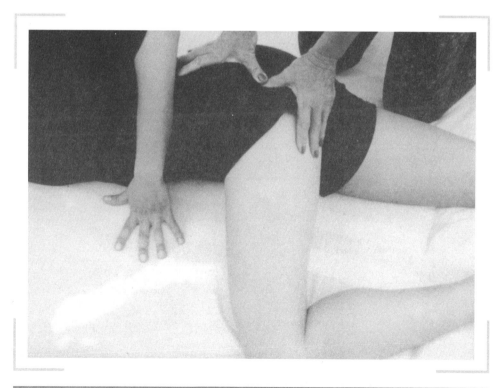

Exercise 89

The patient lies on his side.
The practitioner sits on his knees behind the patient's back.
The massage is performed in the region of the back, from the pelvis in
the direction of the shoulders, applying walking P.P. back and forth.

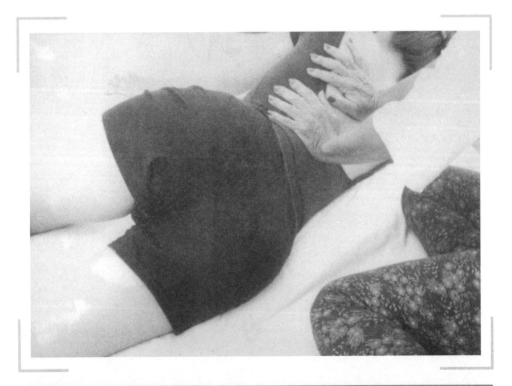

Exercise 90

The patient and the practitioner are in the same position.
The massage is performed by T.P., alternately, five seconds on each
treatment point, back and forth. The pressures are applied on both sides
of the spine, along the two energy lines.

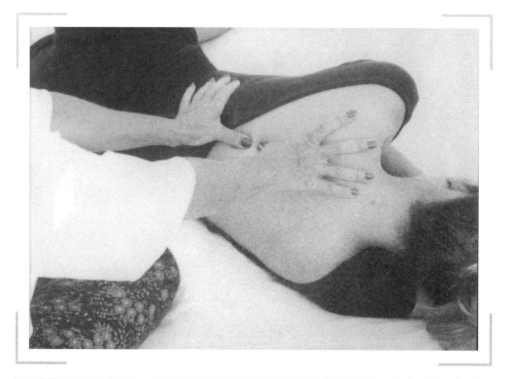

Exercise 91

The patient and the practitioner are in the same position.
The massage is performed on the whole back by P.P., alternately, several times, back and forth, for relaxation.

Exercises 75-91 are repeated on the other leg and on the other side of the patient's back.

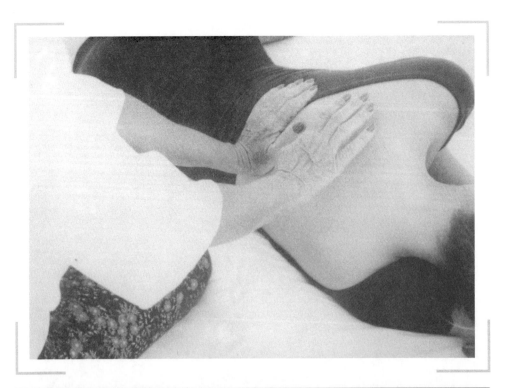

Exercise 92

The patient sits, one knee bent, his arms hugging it.
The practitioner kneels behind the patient.
The practitioner grasps the patient's shoulder (on the same side as the bent knee) with both hands, fingers interlaced. The practitioner's arm is under the patient's armpit, pulling, pressing, and moving alternately, three times.

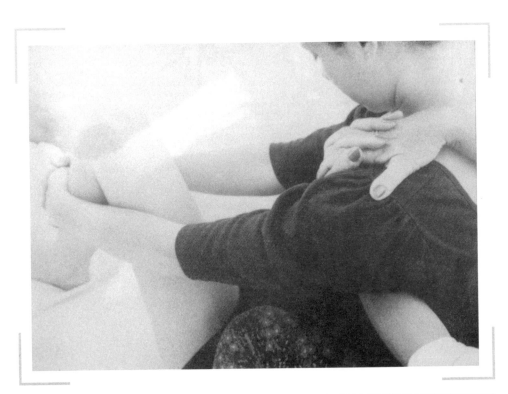

Exercise 93*

The patient lies on his side.
The practitioner sits behind the patient.
One of the patient's arms is raised above his head, while the other lies straight on the floor.
One of the practitioner's knees supports the shoulder-blade of the patient's raised arm, while his other knee is on the floor.
With one hand, the practitioner holds the patient's raised forearm above the wrist, and with the other hand, presses on the patient's armpit, and performs stretching.

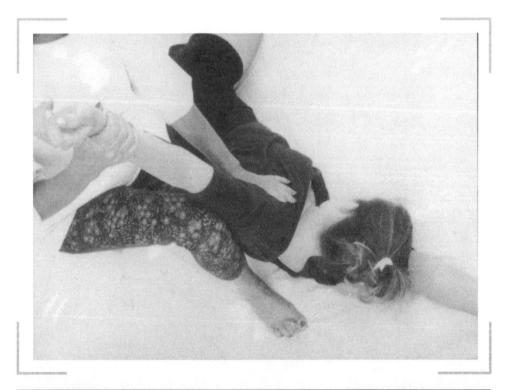

Exercise 94*

The patient lies on his side.
The practitioner stands behind the patient's back.
The patient rests his head on his forearm, which points behind his head at a right angle, crossing his other hand.
With one hand, the practitioner holds the outstretched arm in the region above the wrist, and with the other, grasps the shoulder of the opposite arm, and performs stretching.

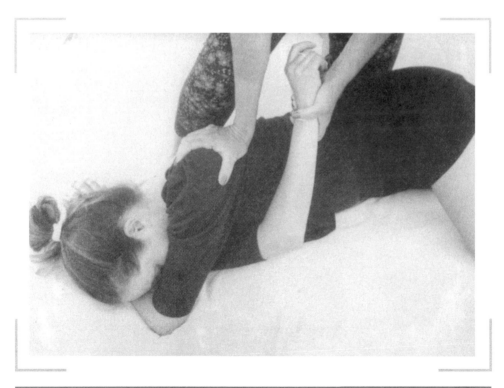

Exercise 95*

The patient and the practitioner are in the same position.
The patient's right arm is on the floor, at a right angle to his body, and his right leg is straight.
His left hand is on the floor, on the same side as his right arm.
With his left knee on the floor, the practitioner supports the patient's left leg in the region of the thigh bone. The practitioner raises this leg and brings it close to his own left shoulder, holding it in the area of the calf. With his other hand, the practitioner holds the patient's left shoulder, and performs stretching.

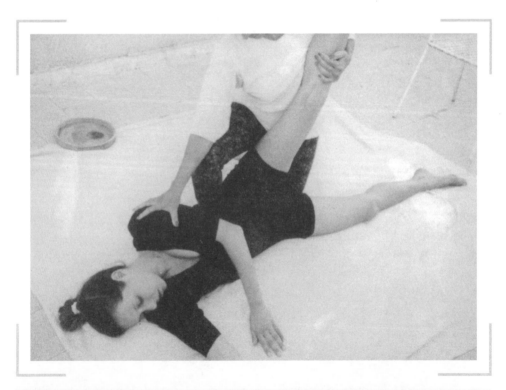

Exercise 96*

The patient and the practitioner are in the same position.
The patient's left leg is bent over his right leg, and rests on the floor.
The practitioner supports the patient's back in the area of the waist with
his right knee. With his right hand, he holds the patient's right shoulder,
and with his left hand, he holds the patient's bent leg, in the area of the
pelvis, and performs stretching.

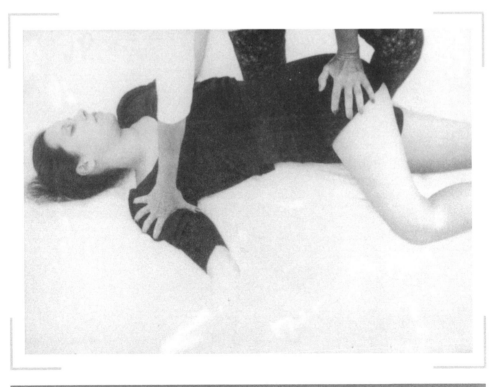

Exercise 97*

The patient lies on his stomach.

The practitioner stands.

With one hand, the practitioner holds the patient's hand above
the region of the wrist, and with the other hand, he holds the patient's
opposite leg, which is lifted.

One of the practitioner's legs supports the patient's back in the region
of the waist, while the other foot is placed on the patient's back
in the region of the waist.

The practitioner performs stretching and pressing of the region
of the lower back three times.

The practitioner repeats the exercise with his other leg.

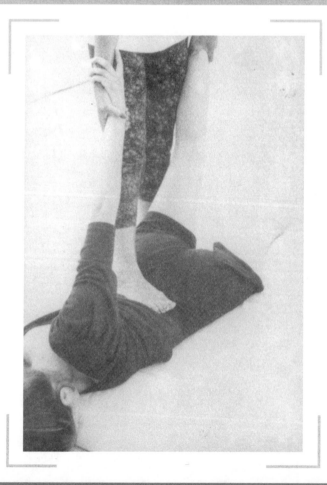

Exercise 98

The patient lies on his stomach, with his legs slightly apart.
The practitioner stands.
Standing with his back to the patient, the practitioner places
the soles of his feet on the soles of the patient's feet,
and applies pressure with his heels three times.
The practitioner turns around, facing the patient's head,
the soles of his feet on the soles of the patient's feet,
and applies pressure with his heels three times.

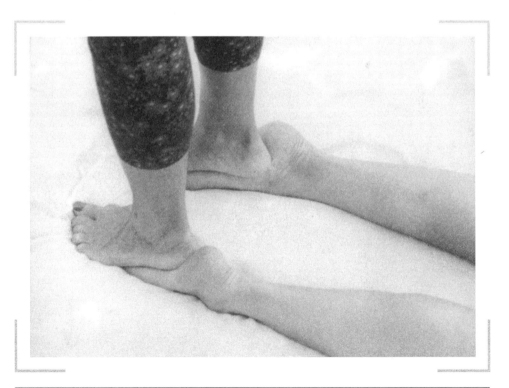

Exercise 99

The patient and the practitioner are in the same position.
The patient bends one of his legs at a right angle.
One of the practitioner's knees is on the floor, the other upright in front
of him. The patient places the back of his foot on the practitioner's
upright knee. With one hand, the practitioner massages the sole
of the patient's foot with his forearm, and performs sliding,
while with the other hand, he grasps the patient's raised foot
in the area above the ankle.

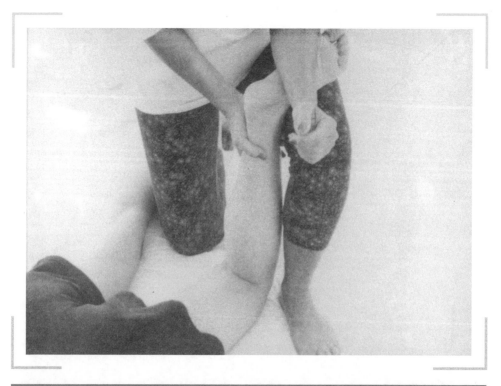

Exercise 100

The patient and the practitioner are in the same position.
The practitioner applies pressure to the six treatment points on the sole of the patient's foot (see the diagram of the foot in the Introduction) with his elbow. The pressures are back and forth, and finally sliding massage is performed.

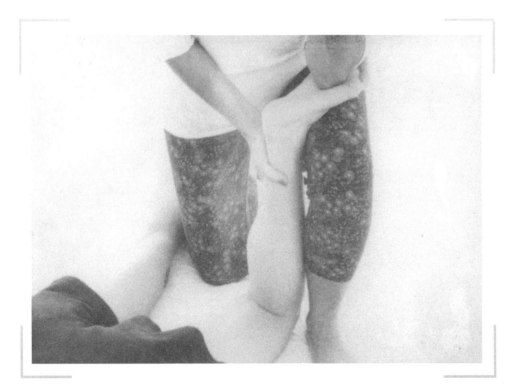

Exercise 101

The patient and the practitioner are in the same position. The practitioner puts the patient's foot down and gets into a comfortable position for massaging the upper surface of the foot with his thumbs. The massage is performed with pressure and rotation movements. Each pressure takes five seconds, and is applied three times. The practitioner raises the patient's foot slightly, and massages the upper surface of the foot while adhering to the following rules:

a. Massage with rotation movements along the upper surface of the foot from the join toward the tip of the toes, back and forth.
b. Application of pressure along the upper surface of the foot, but not on the bones.
c. Finish with "twisting" movements, three times in each direction.

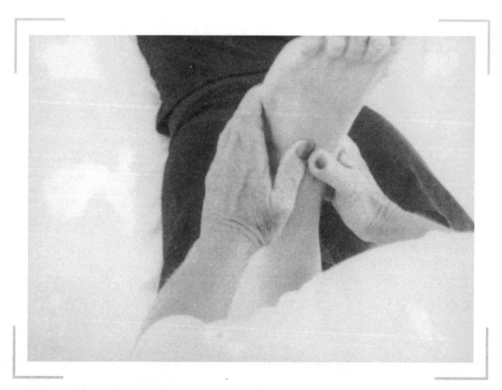

Exercise 102

The patient lies on his stomach.

The practitioner kneels.

The practitioner grasps the upper surface of the patient's foot in his hands, moves it in the direction of the patient's buttocks, and presses three times. He increases the pressure each time.

Exercises 92-102 must be repeated on the other side of the body.

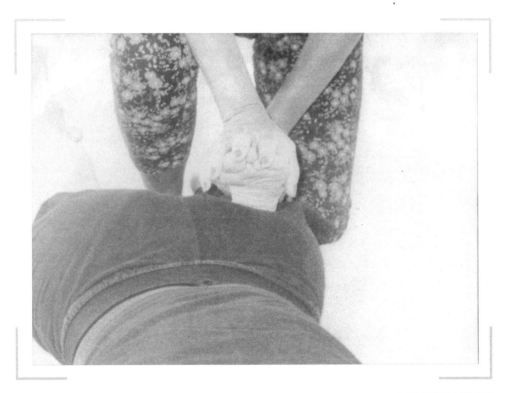

Exercise 103

The patient and the practitioner are in the same position.
The practitioner, who is kneeling behind the patient, crosses the patient's feet and places them on his buttocks, holding them in one hand. With his other hand, he massages one of the patient's legs from knee to ankle, by applying pressure.
The same exercise must be done with the other leg, after crossing the patient's feet the other way.

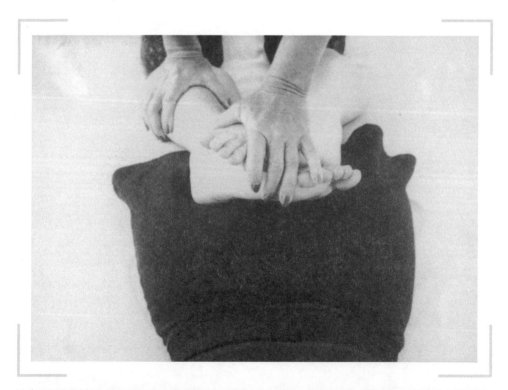

Exercise 104

The patient lies on his stomach, with his hands on the floor, in a
comfortable position. His legs are bent upward, feet touching.
The practitioner leans over him, with his buttocks supported by the
patient's feet (not mandatory).
With both hands, the practitioner massages the patient's back along the
two energy lines at the sides of the spine, applying P.P.
The direction of the massage is from the lower back upward,
pushing the muscle.

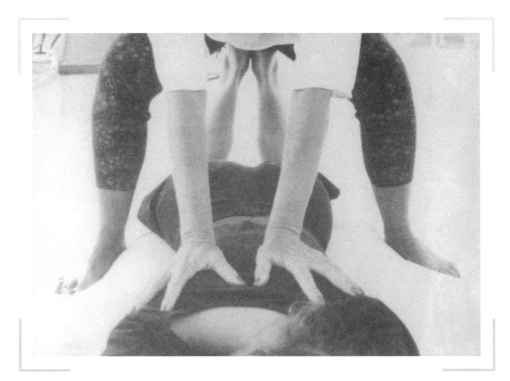

Exercise 105

The patient and the practitioner are in the same position.
The massage is performed using both palms, when most of the pressure
is applied by the two thumbs, which move the muscle in the direction of
the massage, by rotation movements.
(Note the treatment points on the lower and upper back that appear in the
diagram in the Introduction.)

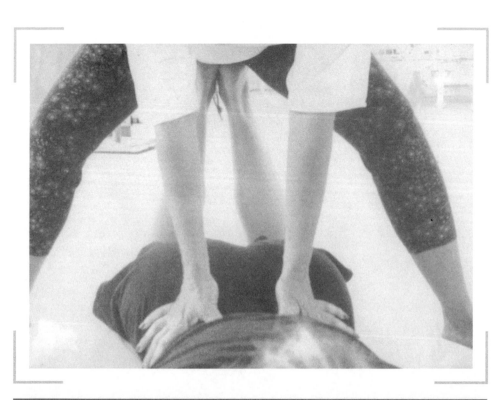

Exercise 106

The patient and the practitioner are in the same position.
The massage is performed by T.P. from the buttocks upward, along the
two energy lines at the sides of the spine. The pressures are applied
alternately by the thumbs, with each thumb moving along
one energy line.

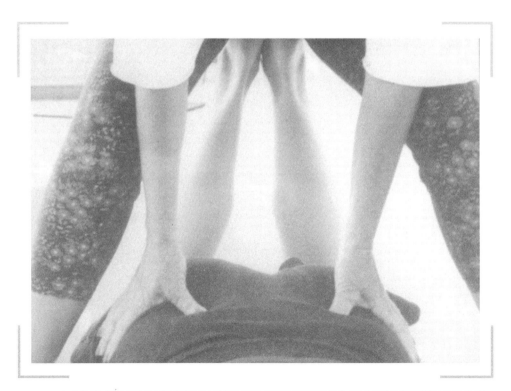

Exercise 107

The patient and the practitioner are in the same position.
The patient's arms rest on the floor, at a 90-degree angle to his body. His legs are bent upward.
The practitioner sits lightly on the patient's feet - as if on a stool - with his own feet on either side of the patient's body, supporting himself. His two hands grasp the front of the patient's shoulders, and he pulls them toward himself three times, progressively higher each time.

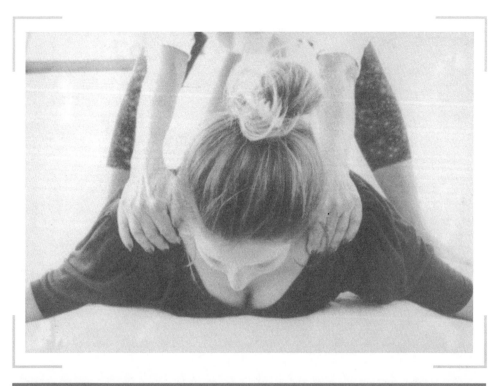

Exercise 108*

The patient and the practitioner are in the same position.
The practitioner interlaces his fingers, and gently lifts one of the patient's shoulders three times, while his foot (on the non-raised of the patient's body) supports the patient's non-raised armpit.
At the second stage, the practitioner rotates the patient's shoulder several times in each direction. The massage is performed with P.P.
The practitioner switches hands and massages the other shoulder.

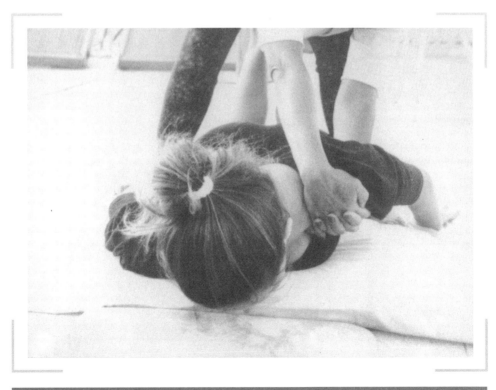

Exercise 109*

The patient lies on his stomach.
The practitioner sits on his knees, which touch the patient's buttocks.
His hands hold the patient's forearms and pull him backward as high as possible. The massage is performed using knee pressures along the three treatment points of the outer thigh. The practitioner places his knees so that they touch the patient's buttocks, point after point, while he pulls the patient's body three times.

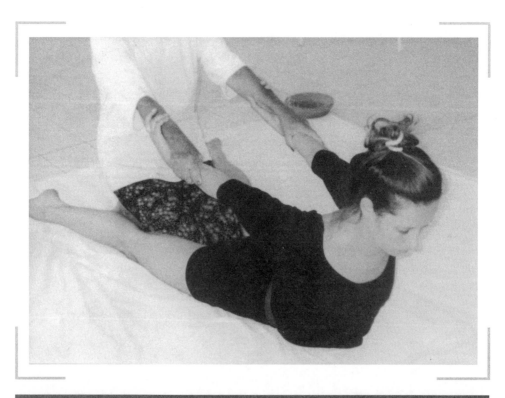

Exercise 110*

The patient lies on his stomach, his legs slightly apart.
The practitioner stands between the patient's legs.
The exercise begins by the application of P.P. on the patient's legs
and back.
Afterward, the practitioner gets up, places one foot on the patient's back,
and applies pressure to the three treatment points, while his other foot
supports the patient's body in the region of the groin.
The practitioner performs the same exercise with his other foot.

Warning! Only qualified practitioners may perform this exercise.

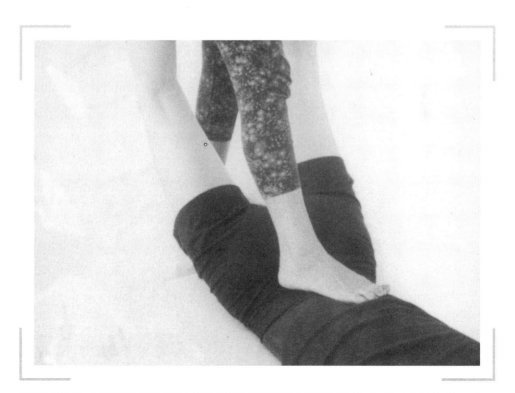

Exercise 111

The patient is in the same position.

The practitioner stands at his side.

The practitioner lifts the arm on the far side of the patient's body, and with his other hand, lifts the patient's diagonally opposite leg, pulling the patient's arm and leg toward himself.

With his foot, the practitioner uses rotation movements to massage the two treatment points on each side of the tailbone.

The exercise is repeated on the other side of the patient's body (other arm/leg).

Finally, the practitioner strokes the patient's back to relax it.

Comment: This exercise is a variation of exercise 97.

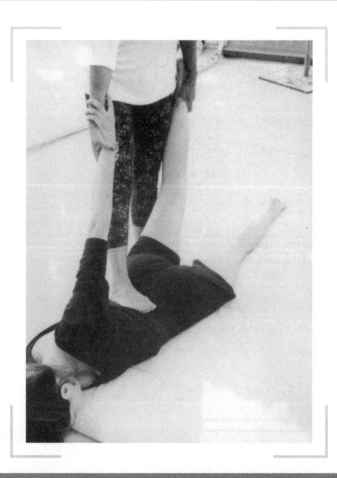

Exercise 112

The patient lies on his back, crosses his legs, lifts them, and leans
them against the practitioner's legs.
The practitioner stands and grasps the patient's forearms.
The practitioner pulls the patient's body toward him three times,
higher each time.
The third time, he sits the patient down cross-legged.

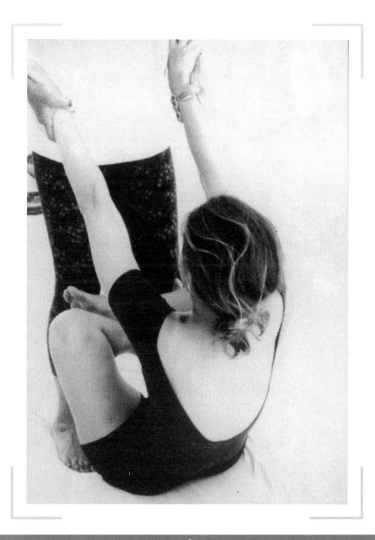

Exercise 113

The patient sits cross-legged, one hand behind his back, the palm facing the practitioner's knee. With one hand, the practitioner pulls the shoulder of the bent hand toward him; with the other hand, he pushes the patient's back in the opposite direction.

The massage is performed on the shoulder only, using P.P.

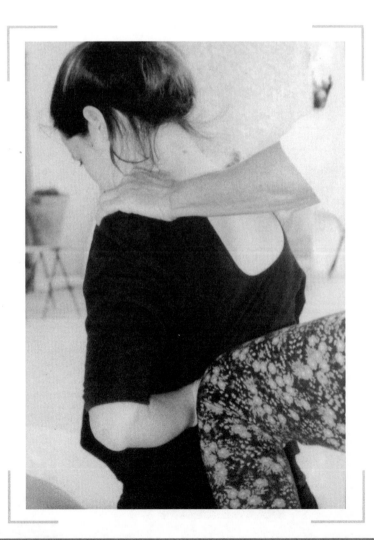

Exercise 114

The patient sits cross-legged.
The practitioner kneels behind him.
The patient's bent arm is lifted backward, and the palm is placed on the practitioner's chest. The practitioner holds this hand in one hand, and uses his other hand to massage the bent hand with P.P., back and forth, several times.

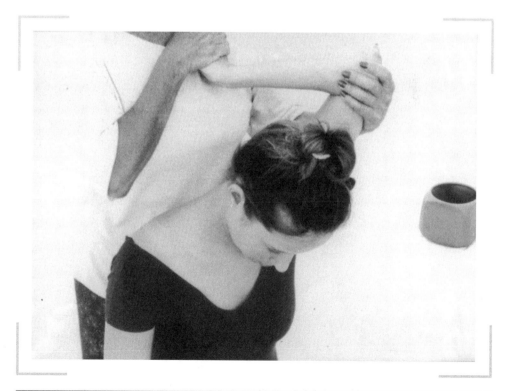

Exercise 115

The patient is in the same position.

The practitioner stands behind him.

The arm that is being worked on is placed close to the back of the patient's neck.

The practitioner holds the patient's bent arm with one hand (close to the elbow). His other hand holds the patient's arm close to the armpit. When the arm muscle is taut, the practitioner pulls the arm toward himself, while his other hand massages the arm using squeezing movements, back and forth, from the armpit to the elbow and back.

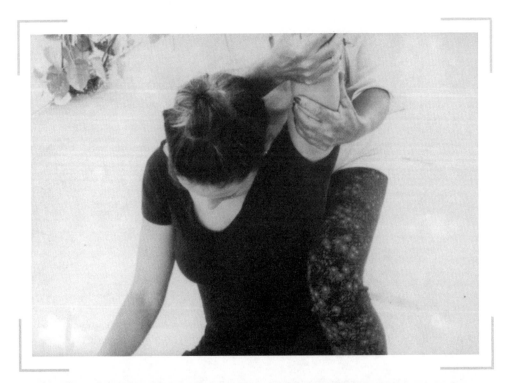

Exercise 116

The patient is in the same position.
The practitioner kneels behind the patient.
The patient's arm is raised and bent backward.
With one hand, the practitioner holds the patient's upper arm, and with the other clenched in a fist, he performs "hitting" back and forth, from the elbow to the armpit and back.

Exercises 113-116 must be repeated with the other arm.

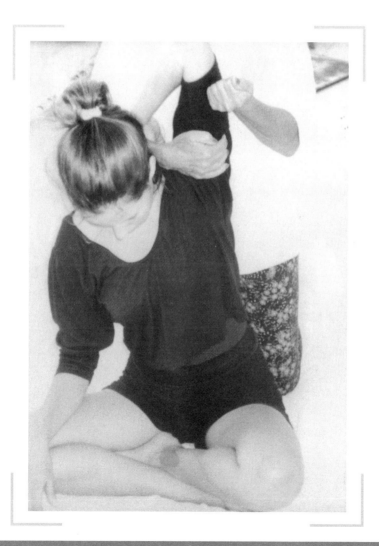

Exercise 117

The patient sits cross-legged (or in another position).
The practitioner stands behind the patient.
The patient's fingers are interlaced behind his head, touching
the back of his neck.
The practitioner gets the patient's arms to touch his body, holding them
in the region of the elbows, and pulls them toward his body three times,
more strongly each time.

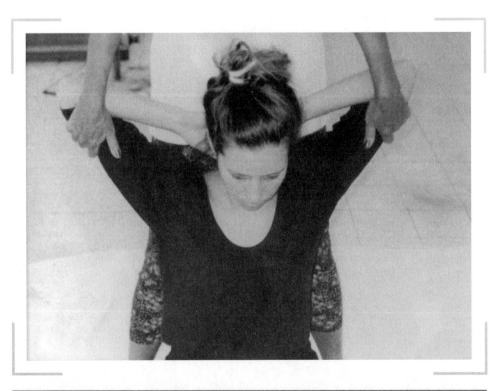

Exercise 118

The patient sits cross-legged.
The practitioner kneels behind him.
The patient's fingers are interlaced, supporting his nape. His elbows
are as far from his body as possible, and lifted upward.
The practitioner's hands hold the patient's forearms from
the inside outward.
The exercise is leaning the patient's body forward, three times,
closer to the floor each time.

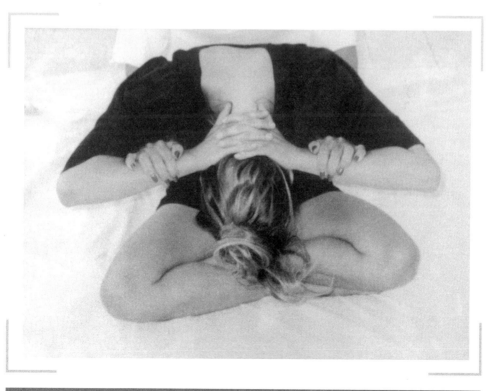

Exercise 119

The patient and the practitioner are in the same position.
The practitioner activates his body weight, in order to make the patient's body lean to the left and to the right, three times on each side.

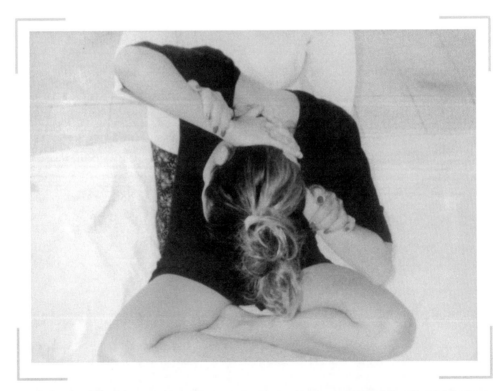

Exercise 120

The patient sits cross-legged (or in another position).
The practitioner kneels behind him.
With fingers interlaced, the practitioner's hands hold one of the patient's shoulders at the armpit. While pressing on the patient's back with his knee, the practitioner pulls the patient's shoulder toward him three times.

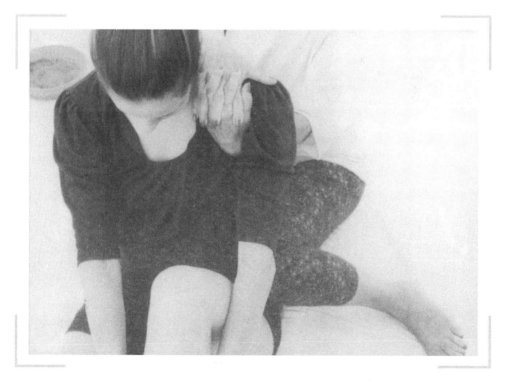

Exercise 121

The patient sits cross-legged. One hand is raised and bent backward.
The practitioner stands behind him.
With one hand, the practitioner holds the elbow of the patient's bent arm,
also supporting the patient's head, and with his other hand, he massages
the patient's upper arm several times by P.P., back and forth, from the
elbow to the armpit and back.

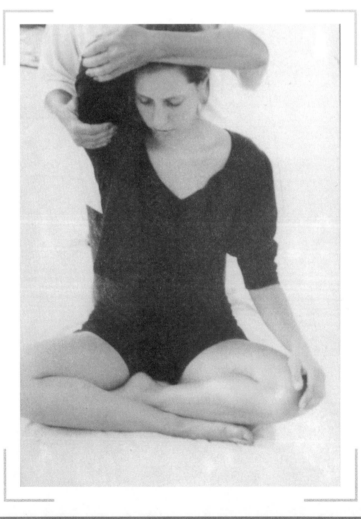

Exercise 122

The patient sits cross-legged.
The practitioner stands behind his back.
With one hand, the practitioner holds one of the patient's shoulders,
while his forearm performs sliding massage on the other shoulder,
back and forth, three times.
Afterward, pressure is applied to the treatment points
on the shoulders with the elbow.

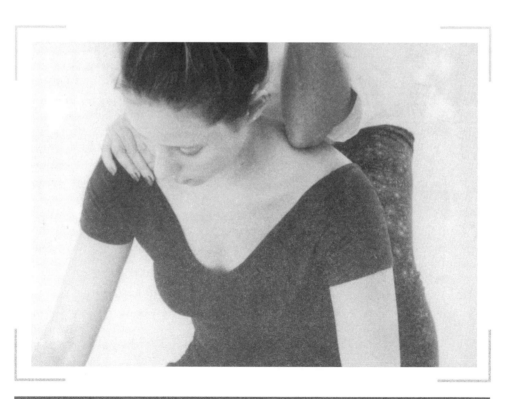

Exercise 123

The patient and the practitioner are in the same position. The practitioner holds the patient's head with one hand, and leans it slightly over to the side. With the elbow of his other arm, he applies pressure to the three treatment points on the shoulder. Afterward, the practitioner performs the sliding movement again.

Exercises 120-123 are repeated on the other side of the body, upper arm + shoulder.

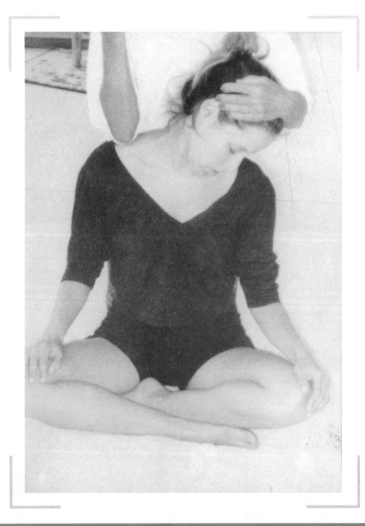

Exercise 124

The patient and the practitioner are in the same position.
The practitioner interlaces his fingers, places them on the patient's nape, and bends the patient's head forward and downward.
The massage is performed by pressure of the pads of the hands on the patient's nape, from the back in the direction of the head, back and forth, three times.

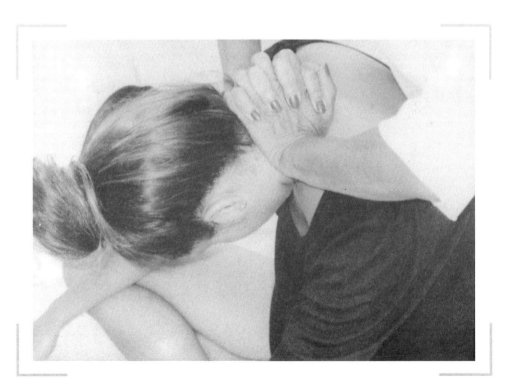

Exercise 125

The patient and the practitioner are in the same position.
The practitioner applies T.P., back and forth, on the patient's nape, with interlaced fingers.
Finally, additional P.P. is applied.

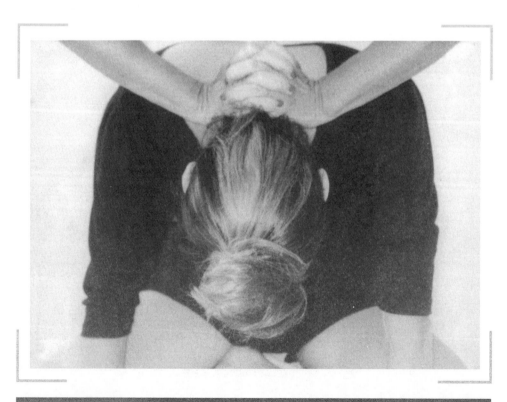

Exercise 126*

The patient sits cross-legged.

The practitioner sits behind him.

The practitioner's feet touch the middle of his back.

His hands grasp the patient's hands, which are stretched backward, in the area of the forearms.

The practitioner performs "walking" with his feet on the patient's back, while pulling his arms toward him, and then he applies pressure to the three treatment points on the lower back with his feet.

The pressure can be applied by the knees instead of the feet.

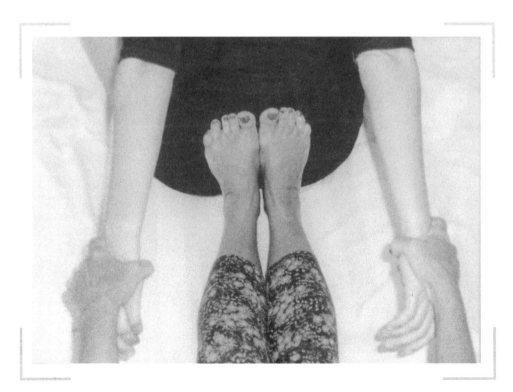

Exercise 127

The patient sits cross-legged.
The practitioner kneels behind him.
The patient's hands are relaxed on the floor or on his knees,
his head bowed.
The massage is a general massage of the back, which starts with P.P. on
the whole back, and continues with T.P. along the two energy lines at the
sides of the spinal column. The massage is performed pushing the
muscles upward.

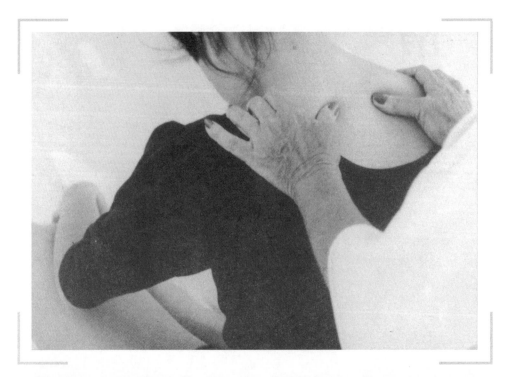

Exercise 128

The patient and the practitioner are in the same position.
The practitioner performs the massage by squeezing movements in opposite directions along the entire back.
Then he performs P.P. on the whole back, as well as "chopping" massage.
The massage of the back concludes with light stroking movements on the whole area of the back and the shoulders.

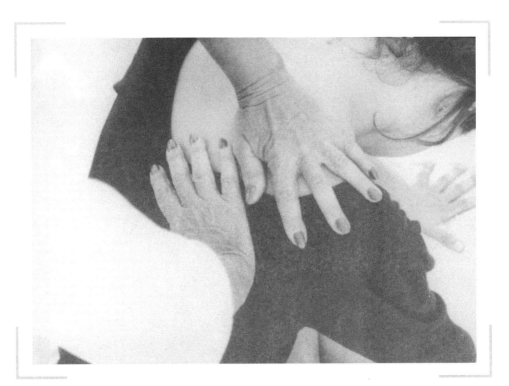

Massage of the Head (Ex. 129-130)

Massage of the head can be performed in two positions: lying down or sitting. (Here we will describe the massage when the patient is sitting cross-legged.) Care must be taken with massage of the head; rotation pressure - not strong - should be applied to all the treatment points.

Exercise 129

The patient sits cross-legged.
The practitioner sits behind him.
The practitioner massages the muscles of the neck and shoulders with rotation movements.
The practitioner holds the patient's head on both sides with both hands, and uses both thumbs to perform the massage. The massage is performed by rotation movements, three five-second pressures on each treatment point. (See the diagram of the treatment points of the head in the Introduction.)

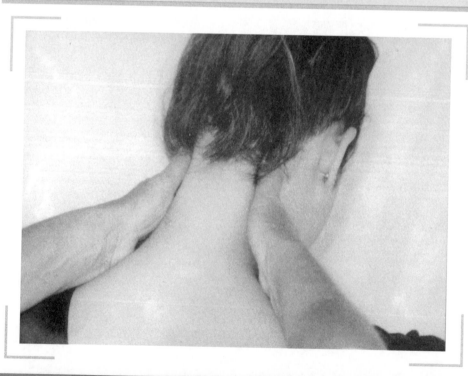

Exercise 130

The patient and the practitioner are in the same position.
The massage of the head begins with three treatment points: The point in the middle of the hollow at the base of the head, and on both sides of the hollow, on the two points that are at the base of the head.
Then the points in the region of the ears are massaged, using T.P. for five seconds as well as turning movements.
The massage of the head ends with "shampooing" movements in all directions. (See the description of the treatment points of the head in the Introduction.)

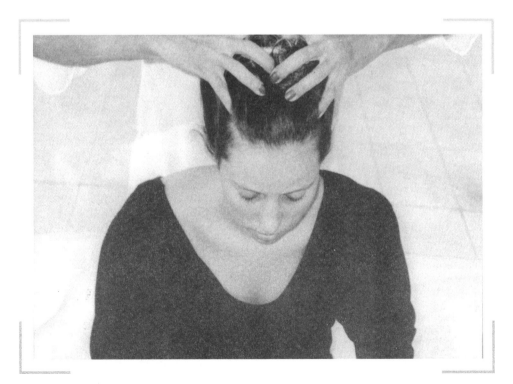

Massage of the Face (Ex. 131-135)

Exercise 131

The patient sits cross-legged.
The practitioner kneels or stands behind him.
The practitioner holds the patient's chin between his interlaced fingers,
and lifts the patient's head gently, bending it to the right and left.
The patient's head is held between the practitioner's forearms.
During the bending of the patient's head, the practitioner lightly
massages the region of the patient's chin.

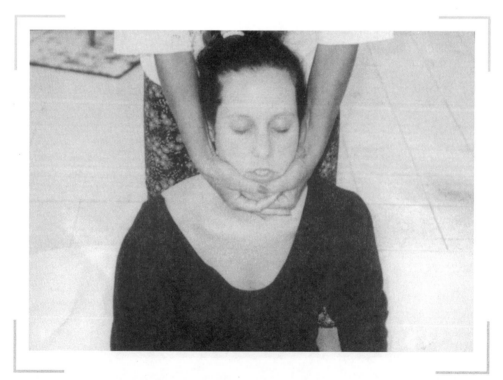

Exercise 132

The patient and the practitioner are in the same position.
The starting point of the massage is in the center of the forehead (the "third eye").
The massage is performed by both thumbs, one on top of the other, using pressure and rotation movements, point after point.
The practitioner massages from the center of the forehead toward the nose, and continues along the eyebrows, on three points. (See the diagram of the face in the Introduction.)

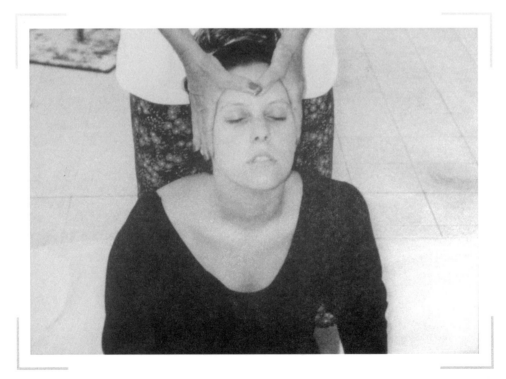

Exercise 133

The patient and the practitioner are in the same position.
The practitioner's hands hold the patient's chin. Using both thumbs, he applies light pressure on the region of the tear ducts - five seconds for each pressure, three times.

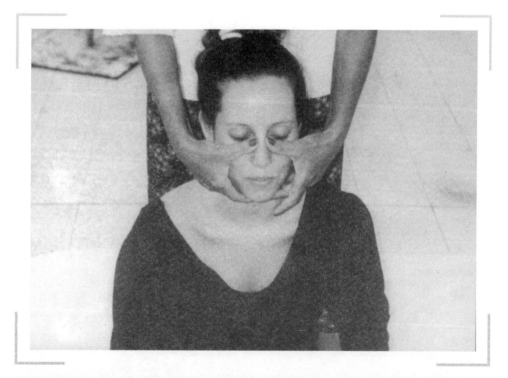

Exercise 134

The patient and the practitioner are in the same position.
The practitioner massages the patient's face with the pads of his fingers,
using rotation movements, starting at the temples and going down.
This massage should be repeated several times.
Afterward, the practitioner applies T.P. in the region of the temples, five
seconds for each pressure, and rotation movements after each pressure.

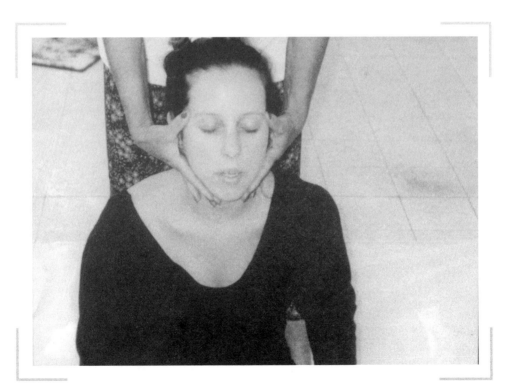

Exercise 135

The patient and the practitioner are in the same position.
The practitioner holds the patient's earlobes between his fingers, rubs them gently, and pulls them downward several times.

After the massage of the face, the practitioner strokes the patient's face alternately from the chin outward.

At the end of the whole massage, pressure must be applied to the "third eye."
The practitioner opens his hand and holds the patient's face, his fingers supporting his head under the chin, his thumbs pressing the "third eye" point. The massage of this point should continue for a few seconds, and is then repeated several times.

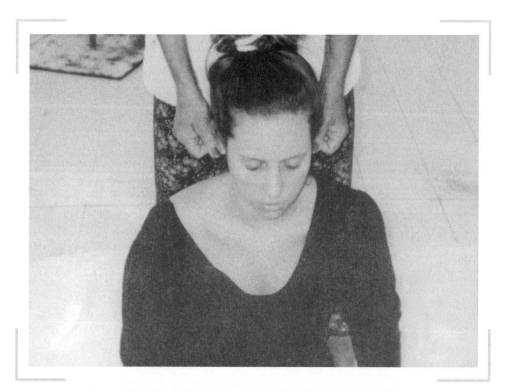

"DO-IT-YOURSELF!" – SELF-MASSAGE EXERCISE PROGRAM

It is possible to perform most of the exercises of Thai massage on oneself. That is, the person massages himself, following the basic rules for treatment.

This part of the book will fulfill the needs of those people who are interested in learning and understanding the basic principles of this self-massage.

The basic principle is that Thai massage is pleasure, not suffering, and therefore it should be performed gently, considerately, and not by force.

Self-massage is important not only for people who are interested in treating themselves, but also for those who treat others, so that they feel on their own body both the energy lines and the power of the palms and thumbs (which are the main "tools") in the pressures and stretching.

A person who performs exercises on himself first finds the most comfortable position for himself, and sometimes improves it over time. Every massage begins and ends with relaxation, a quiet atmosphere, and pleasant background music, without external disturbance, if possible. The person chooses one of the following positions, according to the conditions of the place, his body structure, and the exercise.

- A. Seated on an armchair with broad armrests, for supporting the leg or the arm that is being treated.
- B. Seated on the floor, his back leaning against a wall or piece of furniture.
- C. Lying on his back (for certain exercises).
- D. Lying on his stomach (for certain exercises).
- E. Lying on eiher side (for certain exercises).
- F. Standing (for certain exercises).

It goes without saying that if a particular exercise causes discomfort or pain, it must be stopped, and not repeated. Having said that, in specific cases of knee, neck, head, back, or shoulder pains, almost every exercise will cause mild pain, but it must be repeated in order to attain good results.

In cases of strong muscle cramps, it is a very good idea to warm the place with a warm towel before the massage, in order to relax.

It is highly recommended to use a hot-tub or a sauna before the massage, in order to attain muscle relaxation, increased blood flow, and increased energy flow.

Finally, Thai massage is part of a way of life that includes correct nutrition, a high awareness of inner needs, and the ability to separate oneself from unwanted external influences.

Everyone can.

Everyone must want to do that.

Everyone is capable of doing that.

Everyone owes it to himself:

"Learn to know how and where to touch."

Exercise 1

Sit on the floor or on the bed, legs apart.

Massage both legs simultaneously using alternate palm pressure.

When your hand applies pressure to one leg, your other hand must be in the air, and your body must lean toward the hand that is pressing.

The pressures start at your foot, in the direction of your groin, and back, using "walking" movements. (Don't apply continuous pressure to the area of your knee.)

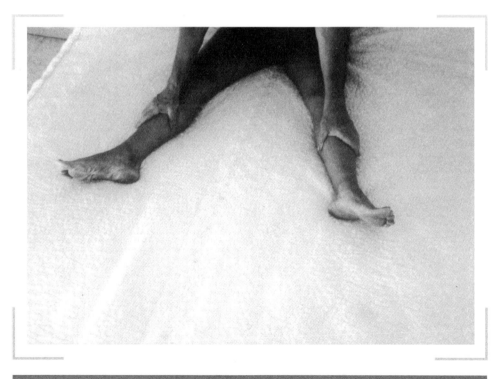

Exercise 2

Sit in the same position.
The massage is a rotation movement in the region of the knees,
simultaneously on both knees, several rotations in each direction. The
massage is performed with an open hand, the center of the palm
on the kneecap.

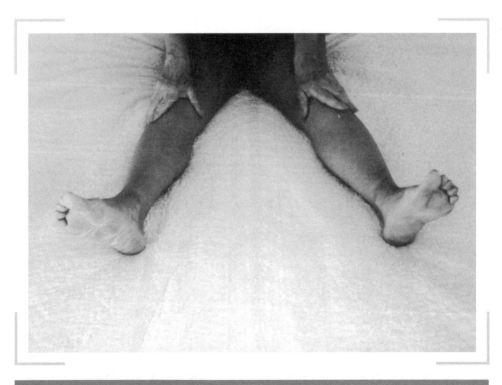

Exercise 3

Move your feet closer to each other, and apply thumb pressure simultaneously on the treatment points on the soles of both feet (see Introduction). While applying pressure with the thumbs, the other fingers grasp the upper surface of the foot and apply gentle pressure to it.

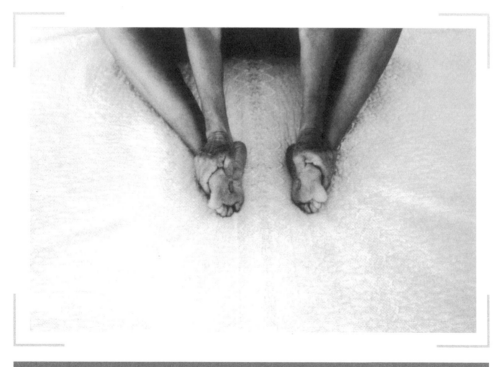

Exercise 4

Place one foot on the other leg, below the knee, so that the foot is outward. (The angle of the bent leg is about 60 degrees.)
Place your thumbs one on top of the other and apply pressure to all the treatment points on the sole of the foot, five seconds per pressure.
After applying the pressure, massage the same place with the thumbs, using rotation movements.

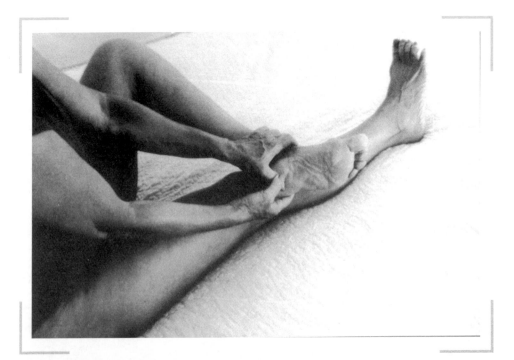

Exercise 5

One leg is straight, resting on the floor, the other is bent at a 30-degree angle (with the knee up).

Using your thumbs, one on top of the other, apply pressure to join point A (see Introduction) for five seconds. Afterward, continue massaging with rotation movements.

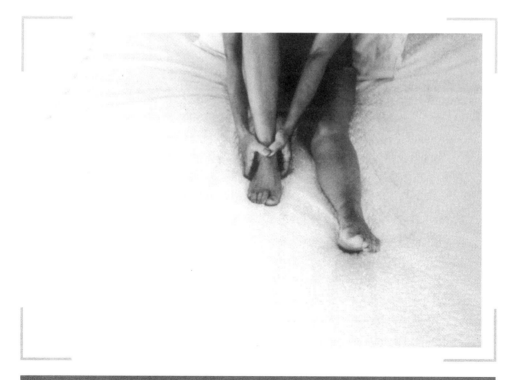

Exercise 6

Sit in the same position, but this time each pair of toes is massaged:
big toe + baby toe, second toe + fourth toe, and the middle toe by itself.
Perform rotation movements from point A in the direction
of the pad of the toe.
Do not apply pressure to the bones, but move the thumbs in the hollow
between the bones, which connect point A to every toe.
Perform the massage back and forth, and when you have finished, gently
pinch the pads of the toes.

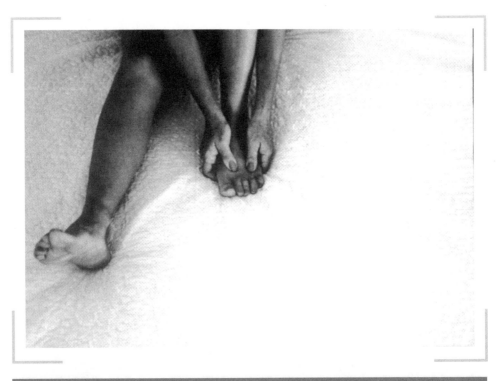

Exercise 7

Bend the leg that is being worked on over the straight leg, without letting them touch. Hold the heel of the leg that is being worked on in one hand, and the toes in the other. Use your thumbs to perform a pressure massage on the treatment points on the muscle of the join (see Introduction). Every pressure lasts five seconds, and is followed by rotation movements by the thumbs.

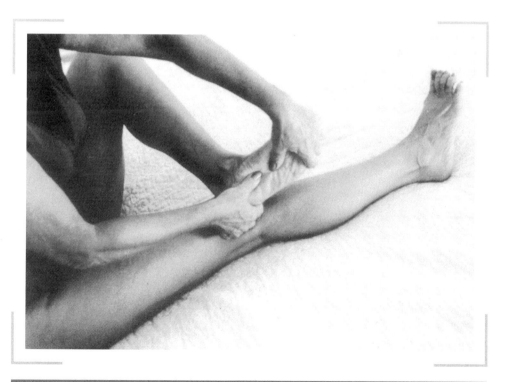

Exercise 8

Sit in the same position. One hand holds the heel of the leg that is being worked on, and the other hand holds both the upper surface and the sole of the foot (in the region below the toes). This hand pulls and turns the foot in the direction of your body, while the other keeps the body stable. Do this exercise 3-4 times.

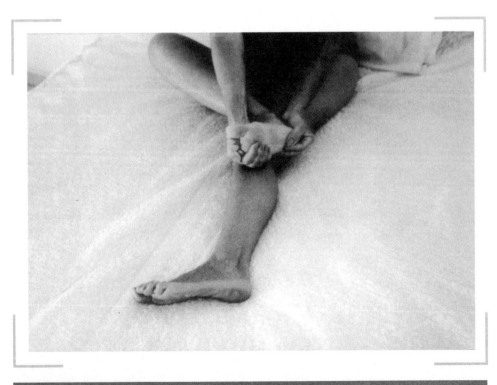

Exercise 9

Massage the sole and the upper surface of the foot that is being worked on with turning movements, using the palms. Then hold the leg that is being worked on in one hand in the region of the ankle, and with the thumb and forefinger of your hand, massage the region of the join of each toe, using rotation movements. After a massage of 10-15 seconds, hold the toe that was treated between your fingers and pull it outward (generally you hear a "cracking" sound).

It is very important that your other hand remains stable while holding the foot.
After you have worked on all the toes, lightly massage the upper surface of the foot with your palms.

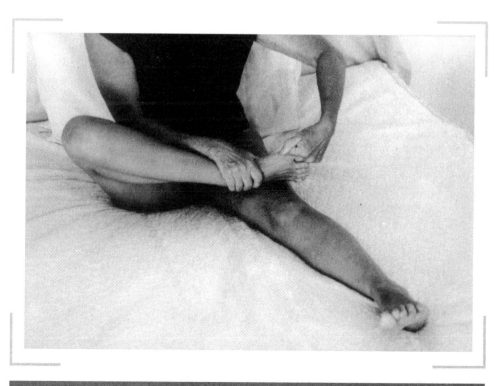

Exercise 10

Bend your leg, knee upward, resting your foot on your straight leg. Apply walking P.P. alternately with both hands along your bent leg, from your toes to your groin, back and forth, three times.

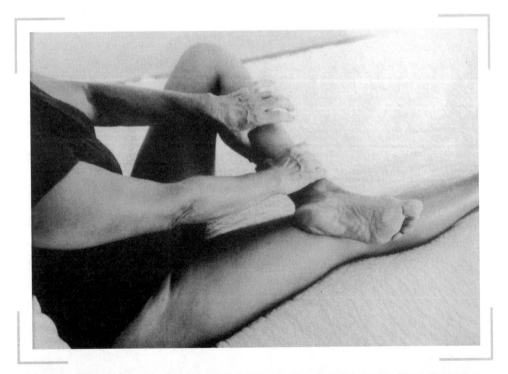

Exercise 11

Sit in the same position. Use your thumbs, back and forth, for massaging energy lines number 1 and 2. Then apply P.P. once, back and forth, on the same place.

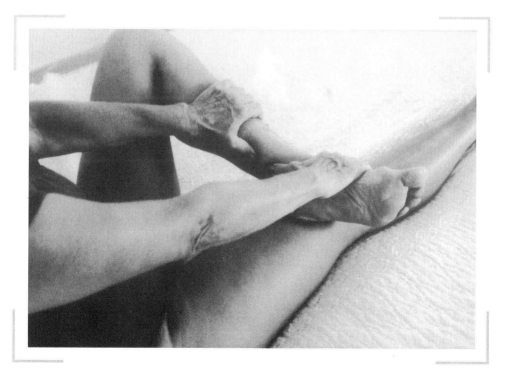

Exercise 12

Sit in the same position. With the center of one hand, hold the heel of the
leg you are working on, keeping your arm straight. With your other
hand, pull your leg in the region of the kneecap, your fingers supporting
your thigh muscle and pulling your leg.
Both hands pull in opposite directions in order to stretch the calf.

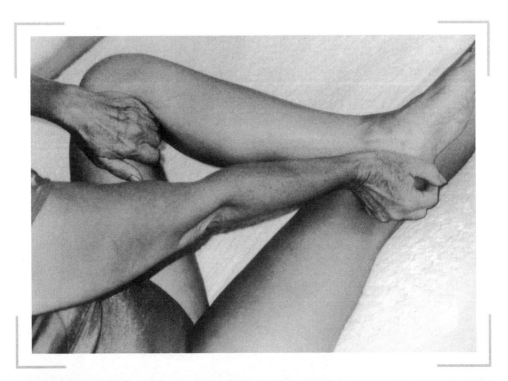

Exercise 13

Sit in the same position. Your bent leg rests on your straight leg below the knee. One hand grasps the thigh of the bent leg (near the knee), and the other grasps the thigh in the region of the groin.
Both hands pull in opposite directions in order to stretch the thigh.

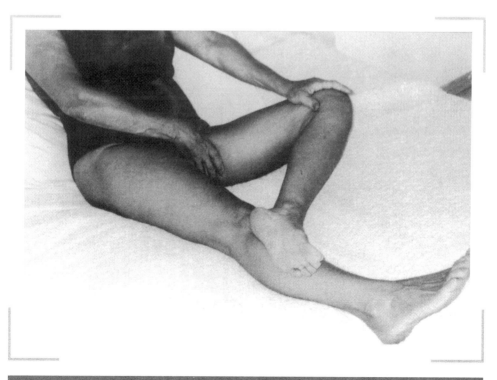

Exercise 14

Sit on the floor, legs slightly apart. Place your hands diagonally one on top of the other, and apply pressure to the groin for 15-30 seconds, for blood stopping.
Perform this exercise once only.

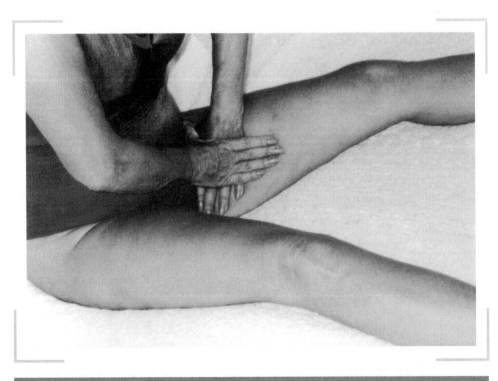

Exercise 15

Sit on the floor or on the bed, your back leaning against the wall. One leg is straight, and the other is bent outward (your knee on the floor). Apply walking P.P. three times to your bent leg, from your foot to your groin.

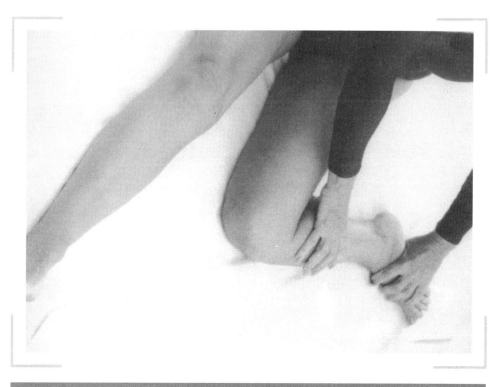

Exercise 16

Apply T.P. once to the leg that is being worked on along outside energy line number 2, back and forth.

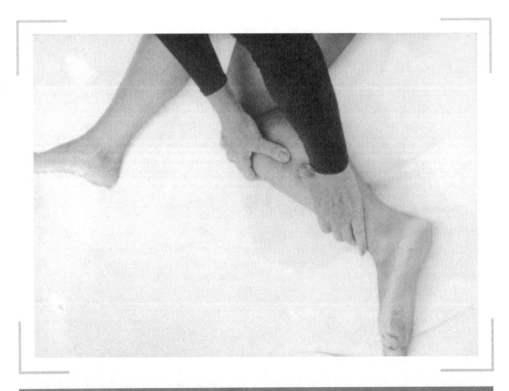

Exercise 17

Apply walking P.P. to the leg that is being worked on alternately, back and forth, from your foot to your groin.
(In the region of the knee, you must change the direction of the palms that are applying the pressure, in order to proceed with the massage comfortably.)

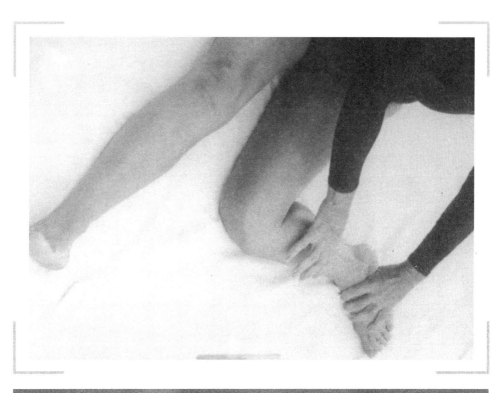

Exercise 18

Place the leg that is being worked on straight out on the floor. One hand grasps the ankle, and the other grasps the knee.
Both hands pull in opposite directions so as to stretch your leg.

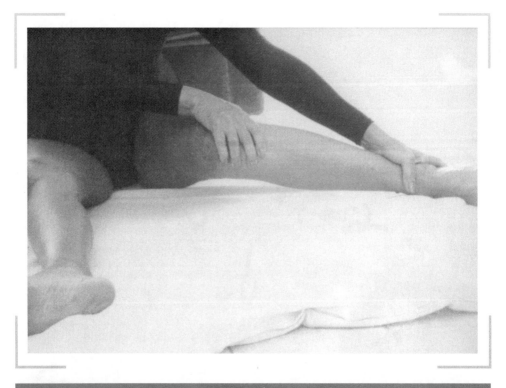

Exercise 19

Bend your leg, with the inner part facing upward. Your other leg is straight out on the floor. With one hand, grasp your straight leg above the knee, and with the other hand, grasp your bent knee. From this position, press on the bent leg three times, harder each time, and try to get it as close to the floor as possible.

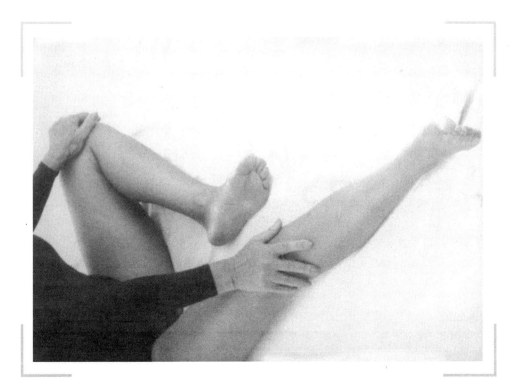

Exercise 20

Lift your bent leg, so that your knee faces upward, and your foot is on the floor (your leg should be bent at a 60-degree angle). Using both hands, apply walking P.P. to your leg alternately, back and forth, from the region of the ankle to the groin, three times.

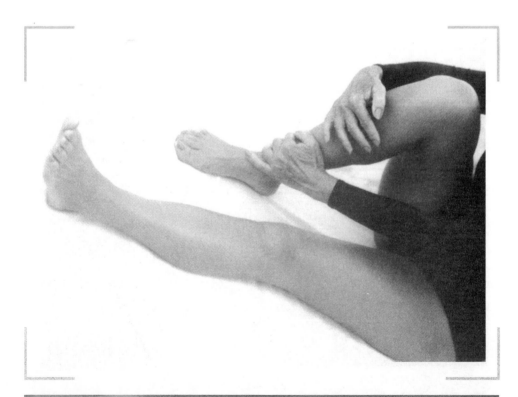

Exercise 21

Sit in the same position. Interlace your fingers around your outer thigh and massage it back and forth, from groin to knee, using the pads of your hands. Then move your thumbs away from each other and apply thumb pressures along the two energy lines (outer and inner) of the thigh, back and forth, once.

End the exercise by applying P.P. on the leg.

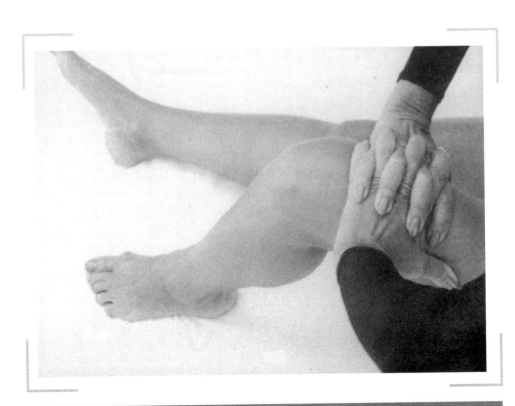

Exercise 22

Sit in the same position. Perform the massage on the inner part of your thigh, applying alternating P.P. and pulling the muscle, back and forth, between the kneecap and the pelvis.

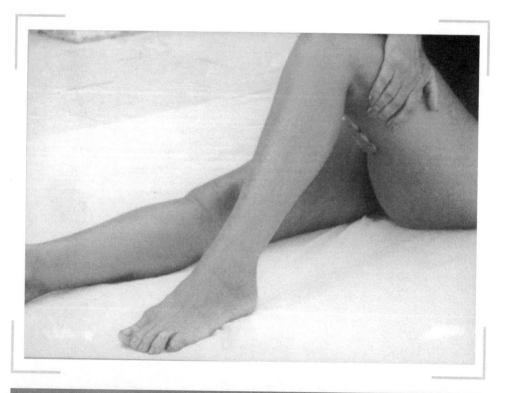

Exercise 23

Sit in the same position. Massage your inner thigh, back and forth, with both your palms, fingers interlaced. Move your thumbs away from each other and apply thumb pressures back and forth, from your kneecap to your pelvis, along the inner and outer energy lines.

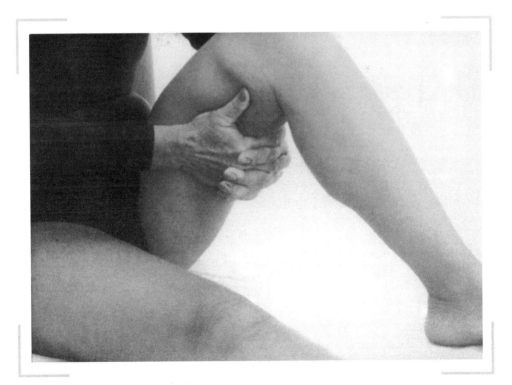

Exercise 24

Sit in the same position. Hold your inner thigh in your hands. Massage it along inner energy line number 3 using the middle and fourth fingers on each hand, from your kneecap to your pelvis, and back. Finish the exercise by applying P.P. and light, releasing slaps to the inner thigh muscle, back and forth.

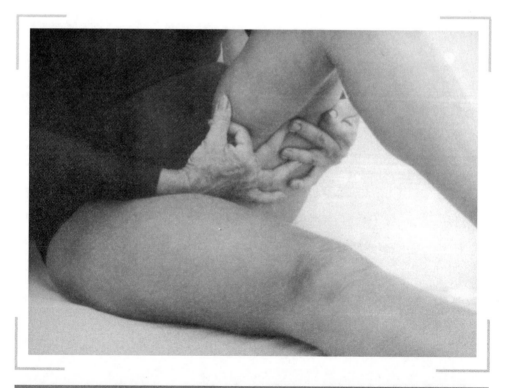

Exercise 25

Sit in the same position, but this time, the angle of your bent leg is narrower. Use P.P. to massage your leg, from your ankle to your kneecap, back and forth along the calf. Then, place your thumbs one on top of the other and massage the inner side of the calf, using pressures and rotation movements (along inner energy line number 3). Finish the exercise by stroking the area lightly, straightening your leg, and placing it on the floor.

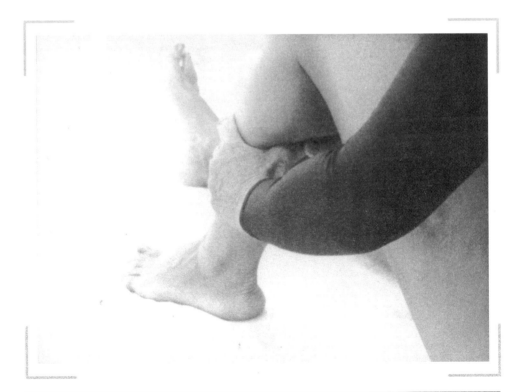

Exercise 26

Bend your leg on the floor, knee inward, and the open angle outward. The other leg is straight out and on the floor.

Place your palms together, and perform "chopping" massage back and forth from the region of the groin to the knee. Both hands strike the leg rapidly but gently.

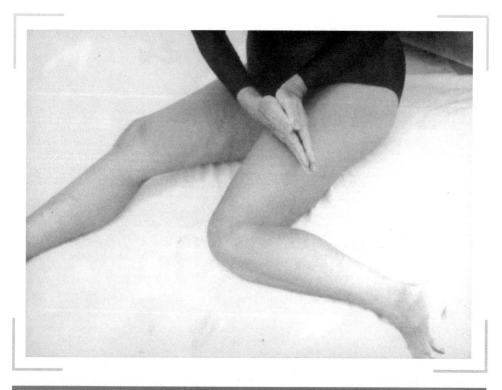

Exercise 27

Sit with your legs straight out on the floor. Lift the leg that is being worked up to a 90-degree angle from the floor, supporting it in both hands. (Before this, you have to bend your other leg so that it supports the knee area of your raised leg.) Pull your raised leg three times toward your body, with straight arms, and get your legs back into the starting position.

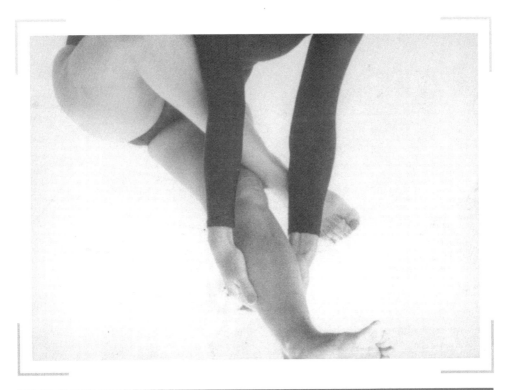

Exercise 28

Repeat the exercise, but this time lying down. Try to bring your raised leg toward your head without supporting it with your arms, while your hands support your body in the area of your waist. At the end of the exercise, put your legs back on the floor, straight out and close together.

Exercises 4-28 are repeated on the other leg.

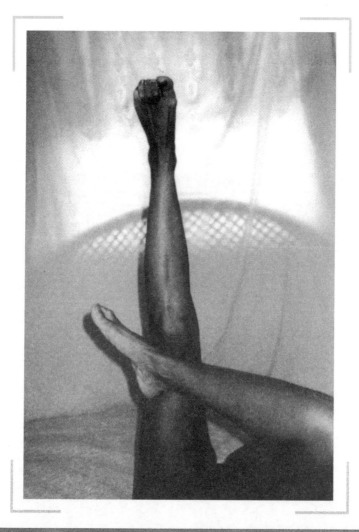

Exercise 29

Lie on the bed or on the floor close to the wall. Clench your fists, and use them to support your lower back. Lift both legs straight and close together toward your head. Using light movements of your clenched fists, you can get your legs to reach the wall behind your head. Do this exercise three times.

At the end of the exercise, unclench your fists and place your legs on the bed or floor to rest.

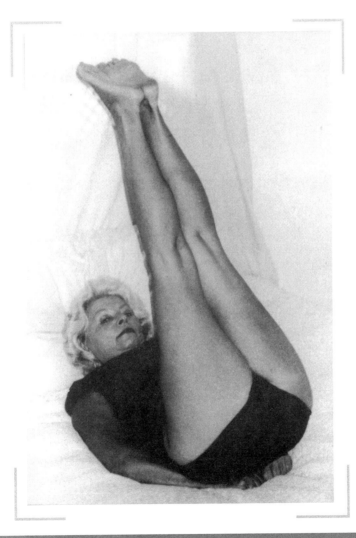

Exercise 30

Sit on the bed or on the floor, your back against the headboard or the wall, both your feet on the floor, and your knees close to each other. (The angle between your thighs and your calves is as small as possible.) Your forearms support your thighs, and your hands grasp your calves, with fingers interlaced.
From this position, lift your legs toward your head three times, as high as possible. At the end of the exercise, straighten your legs and massage them several times, back and forth.

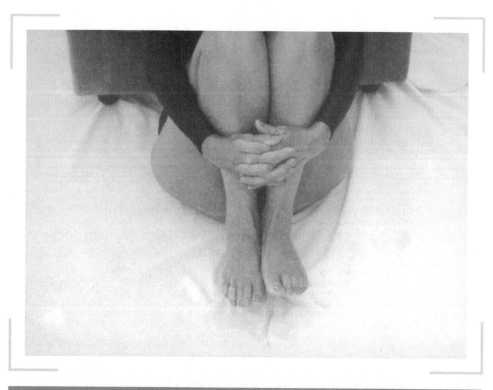

Exercise 31

Sit cross-legged on the bed or floor, your back against the headboard or the wall. Using both hands, hold the upper surface of the opposite foot (right holds left, and vice versa).
Pull your legs upward three times, trying to pull them higher each time. At the end of the exercise, massage the upper surface of your feet with rotation movements.

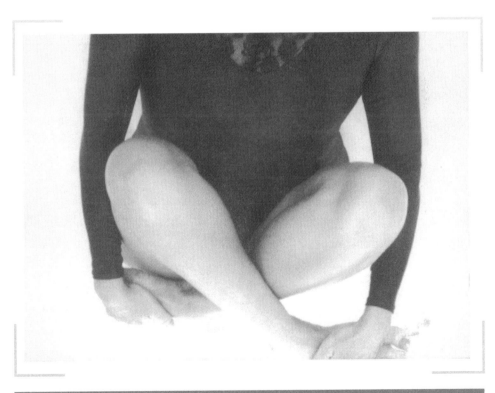

Exercise 32

Lie on your back. Bend your legs, your knees facing your head. With interlaced fingers, hold your calves and pull them hard to your body, three times, pulling harder each time. At the end of the exercise, straighten your legs, shaking them lightly.

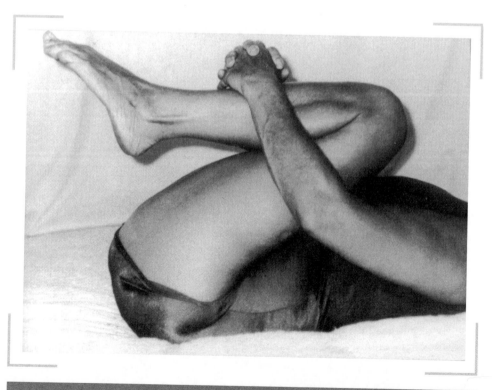

Exercise 33

Lie on your back, your hands stretched out at 90-degree angles at your sides. One leg is straight, the other bent over it at right angles, and your body turns in the opposite direction to the straight leg.
Repeat the exercise, switching legs, and changing the direction of your body.

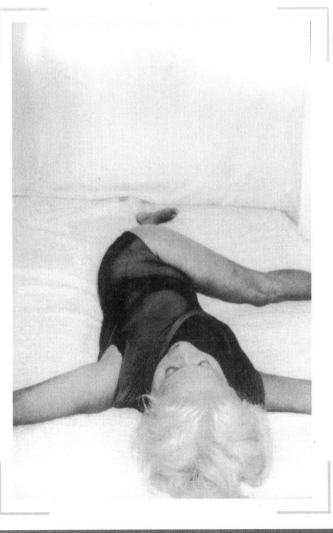

Exercise 34

Lie on your back, one leg straight, the other bent, your knee upward and your foot resting on the thigh of your straight leg. With interlaced fingers, pull your bent leg toward your chest, three times, pulling harder each time.
Switch legs and repeat the exercise with the other leg.

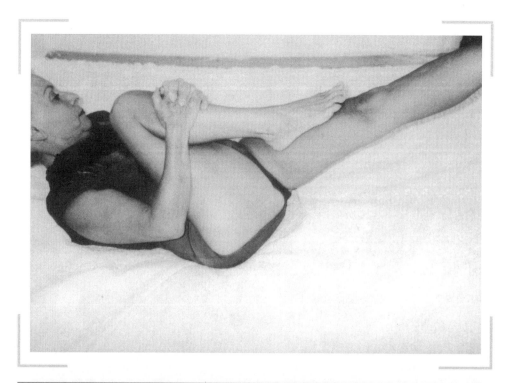

Exercise 35

Sit cross-legged. Hold your knees with your hands. Bend your head
toward the floor and lift it again, three times, your knees close
to the floor.

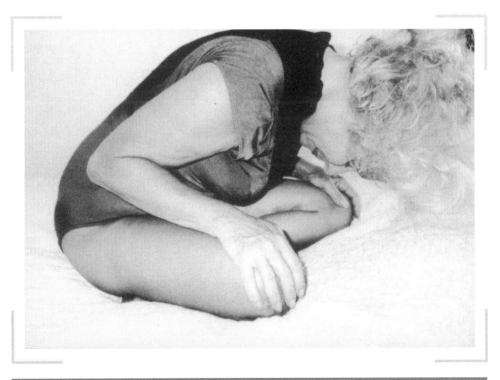

Exercise 36

Sit cross-legged, your feet under your calves (right under left, and vice versa). Using both hands, hold your knees and push them toward the floor three times, pushing harder each time. At the same time, your whole body leans forward and your head gets closer to your legs.
At the end of the exercise, straighten your legs and stroke them, from the toes to the groin and back.

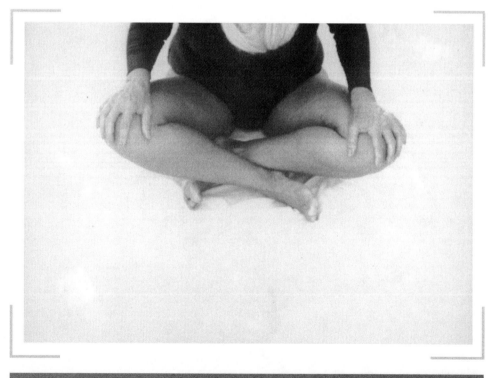

Exercise 37

Lie on your back, your arms stretched straight out on the floor at right angles to your body. One leg is straight, while the other is extended to the side at right angles to your body.

Bring the leg that is extended close to the other leg and stretch them forward. Extend your leg again, and bring it back three times.

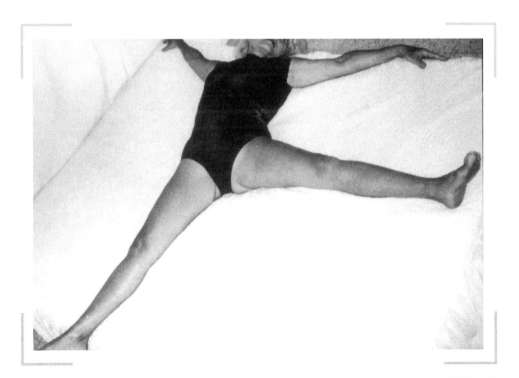

Exercise 38

Lie on your side, one arm on the floor, and your head resting on it. Your other hand is below the armpit of the arm that is straight.
Lift the leg that is on the same side as the bent arm as high as possible. Then lower it onto your other leg. Repeat this exercise three times.

Exercises 37-38 are repeated on the other leg.

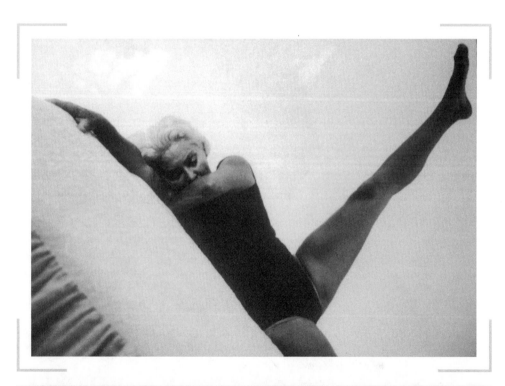

Exercise 39

Comment: Women perform exercises number 39, 40, 41 with raised knees, and men perform them with straight legs, slightly apart.

Lie on your back, your knees raised and your feet on the floor. Apply Rotation Palm Pressure to your whole abdomen, back and forth, in both directions.

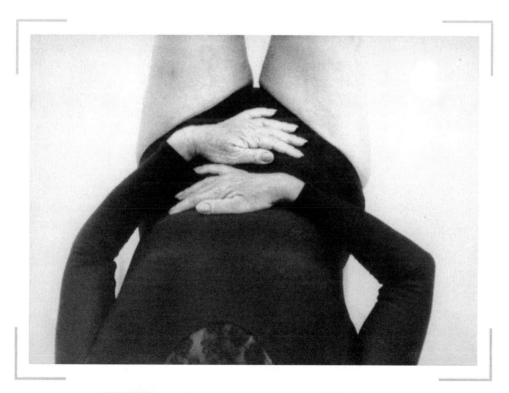

Exercise 40

Lie in the same position. Using both thumbs, apply T.P. to the treatment points on the abdomen (see Introduction). Each time, apply pressure for five seconds to a pair of points, and after each pressure, perform rotation movements with the thumb. During the massage, your hand supports your thigh in the region of the groin, your elbows are far from your body, and your arms lean forward. This position is the one that permits pressure to be applied by the thumbs.

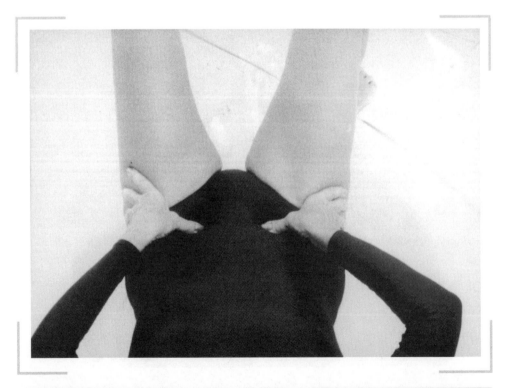

Exercise 41

Lie in the same position. Using both thumbs close together, or one on top of the other, apply T.P. to each treatment point separately, for five seconds. Then apply rotation movements with the thumb. During the massage, your palms support the region close to the point that is being treated, and only the pads of your fingers touch your abdomen.

At the end of the exercise, straighten your legs and massage them several times in order to relax the region of the abdomen and the legs.

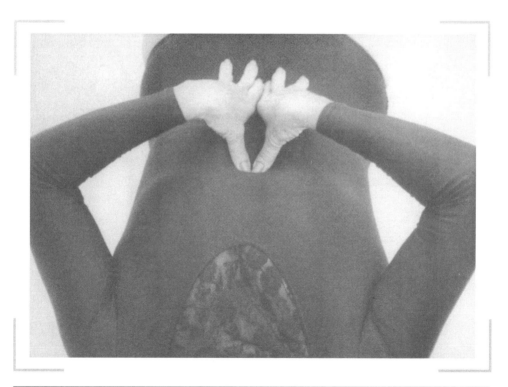

Exercise 42

Comment: The exercises for massaging the arms can also be performed sitting, with the arm that is being worked on supported on an armrest.

Lie on your side. One hand rests on the floor at right angles to the body, with the palm facing upward. Apply P.P. with the other hand, from palm to armpit and back, three times.

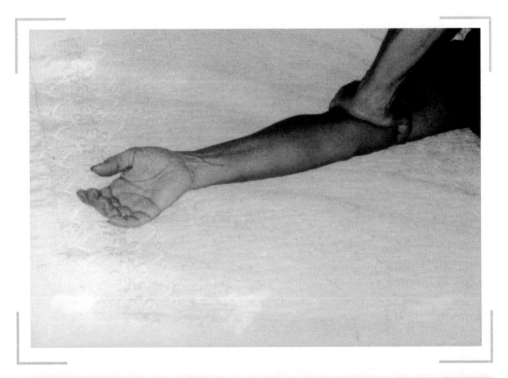

Exercise 43

Lie on your side. One hand rests on the floor at right angles to the body, with the palm facing upward. Using the thumb of the other hand, T.P. is applied, while the rest of the fingers are quite separate from the thumb, and support the arm that is being worked on. The massage is performed along the first and second inner energy lines of the arm
(see Introduction).
At the end of the exercise, massage by P.P., back and forth.

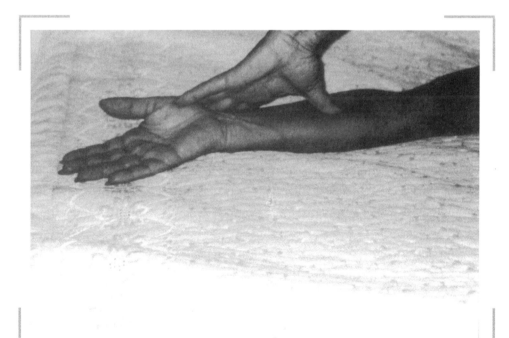

Exercise 44

Lie on your side. Place the arm that is being worked on close to your body, with the upper surface of your hand upward, and your hand resting on your thigh. Perform massage with P.P. back and forth, from palm to shoulder, three times.

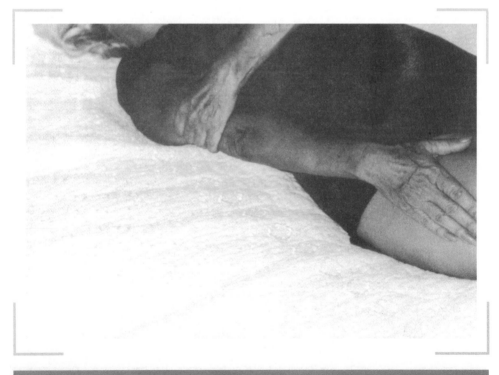

Exercise 45

Comment: Remember that for hand exercises, you should choose the manner of sitting that is most comfortable for you.

Sit on the floor, one leg straight and the other bent over it near the knee, serving as a support for the arm that is being worked on. The forearm of the arm that is being worked on is placed on your bent leg, your hand open palm upward. With the fingers of your active hand, hold the hand that is being worked on, and apply T.P. to the palm (see Introduction). Apply every pressure for five seconds, followed by a rotation movement by the thumb.

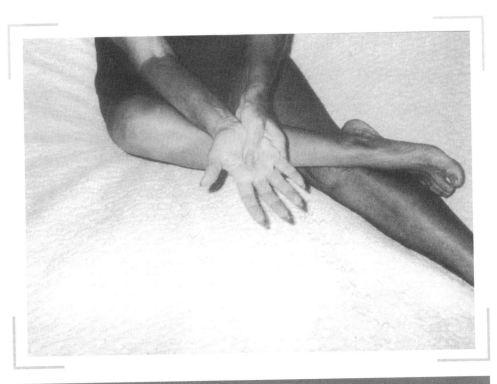

Exercise 46

Sit in the same position. Your active hand massages each finger separately. The massage goes from the wrist to the pad of the finger, several times.
At the end of the massage, pinch the pad of the finger several times.

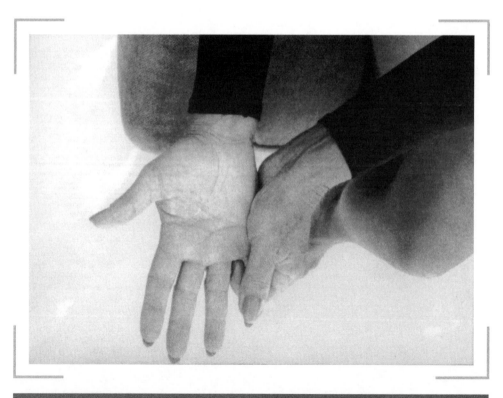

Exercise 47

Sit in the same position. The upper surface of the hand that is being worked on faces upward. The thumb of your active hand applies pressure to the point where your fingers join your wrist (see Introduction). After applying pressure for five seconds, the massage begins with rotation movements along the upper surface of your hand. During the massage, go over the whole area of the hand and fingers, making sure not to apply pressure to the small bones of the upper surface of the hand.

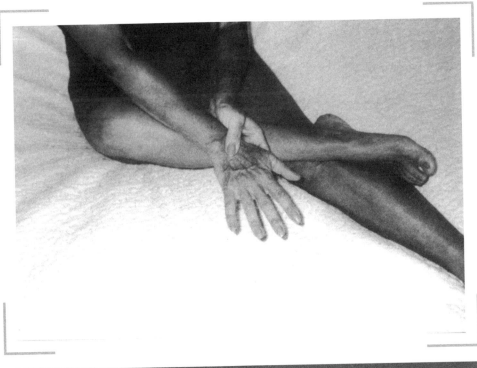

Exercise 48

Sit in the same position. Lightly massage the upper surface of the hand that is being worked on in the region of the join of your fingers to your hand. Use rotation movements, with your thumb above the join and your middle finger below it. The rotation movements are in both directions, several times in each direction. At the end of the massage of each finger, grasp it between two fingers of your active hand, and pull it until a "cracking" sound is heard.

(It is very important that the hand that is being worked on is placed on your leg or on the armrest, for the sake of stability and counterweight.)

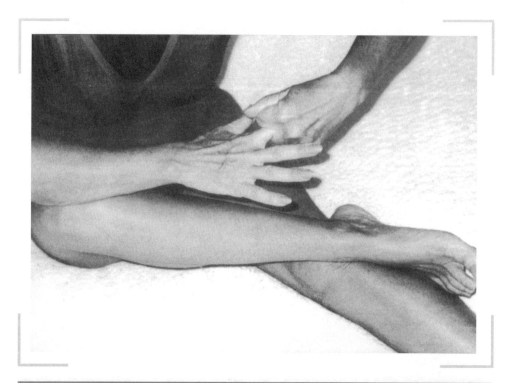

Exercise 49

Sit cross-legged or in any other position that is comfortable for you. Place the hand that is being worked on behind your head, with the elbow upward, your hand touching the back of your head. With the other hand, massage the muscle of your upper arm, back and forth, from the armpit to the elbow, several times.

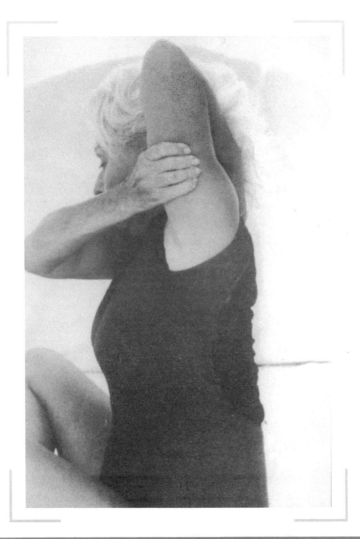

Exercise 50

Apply T.P. along the middle outer energy line, and along inner energy lines number 1 and 2 (see Introduction), from the region of the armpit in the direction of the elbow, and back. Continue applying P.P. in the same region, and end the exercise with light punches in the treatment area.

Exercises 42-50 are now repeated on the other arm.

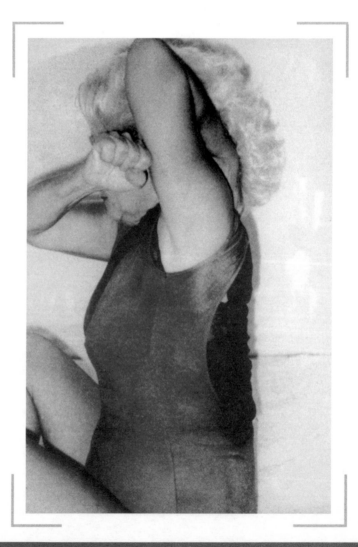

Exercise 51

Sit up straight. Interlace your fingers with your arms facing backward, using them to support the back of your neck.
Use the pads of your hands to massage your neck, back and forth.

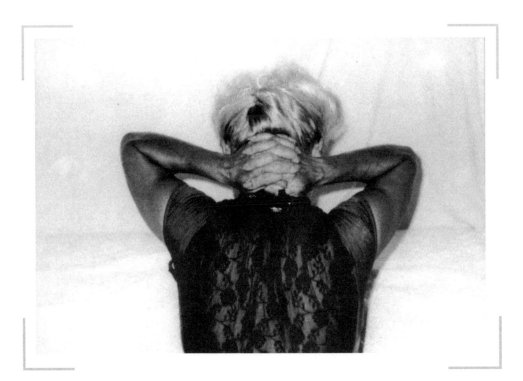

Exercise 52

Sit in the same position, but this time your head is bent forward as much as possible. Place your interlaced fingers on your head, your thumbs pointing downward. Apply T.P. by rotation movements, back and forth, to the region of the treatment points. (It is extremely important to emphasize the rotation movements.)

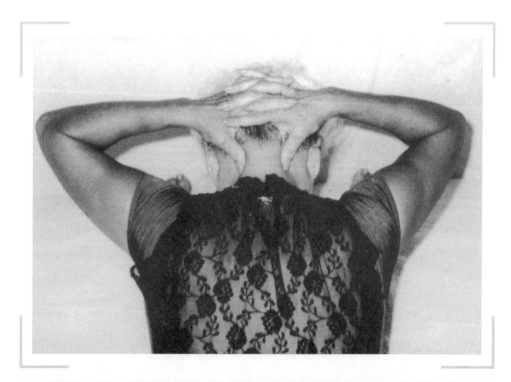

Exercise 53

Sit cross-legged or in any other way that is comfortable for you. Hold the back of your neck with interlaced fingers, applying pressure that causes your head to bend forward, three times, each time nearer to the floor, ensuring that your elbows are close to your body.

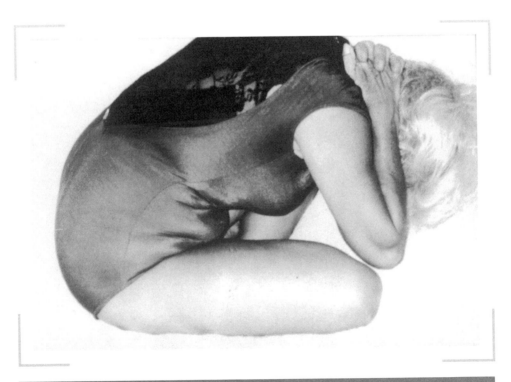

Exercise 54

Sit cross-legged or in any other position that is comfortable for you. The fingers of each hand are close together, and hold your shoulder muscles. Pull your shoulders forward three times, pulling harder each time. Move your hands over the three treatment points on the back of your shoulders (see Introduction).

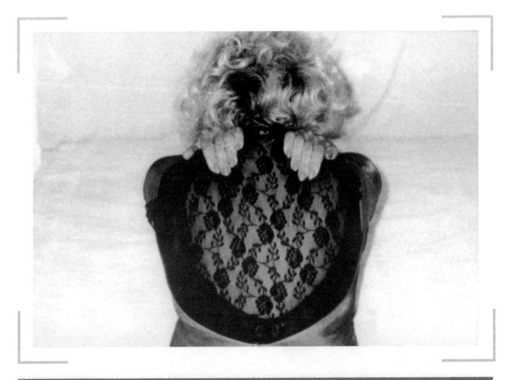

Exercise 55

Repeat the previous exercise with arms crossed: right hand on left shoulder, and left hand on right shoulder.

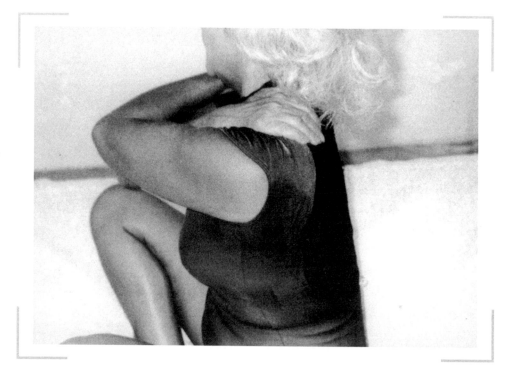

Exercise 56

Sit cross-legged or in any other position that is comfortable for you.
With one hand, hold the shoulder muscle on that arm with closed fingers,
and pull the shoulder forward. Place your other hand over your head,
bending it toward that arm.
The two actions occur simultaneously: pulling your shoulder forward
and bending your head to the side.
Repeat the procedure three times, pulling harder each time.

Repeat the actions with the other shoulder, your head bending
to the other side.

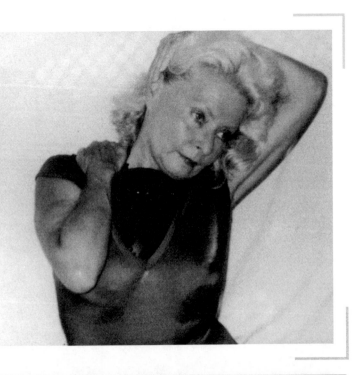

Exercise 57

Lie on your back, legs bent, knees upward. Your interlaced fingers hold the back of your neck, while your elbows point upward, at the sides of your head. By activating the strength in your arms, lift your head three times, higher each time.

At the end of the exercise, straighten your arms and legs.

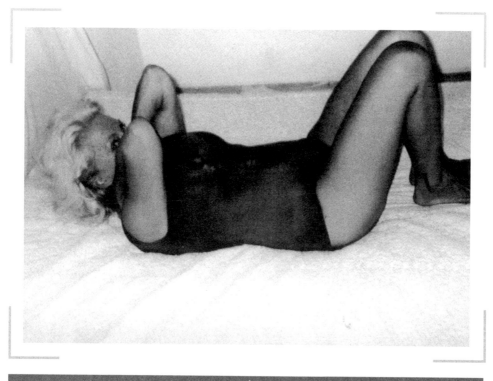

Exercise 58

Sit with your legs straight out in front of you, close together. Your fingers grasp your toes from behind, and pull forward three times. During the exercise, your arms are straight, your head bent downward between your arms, and your legs are straight.

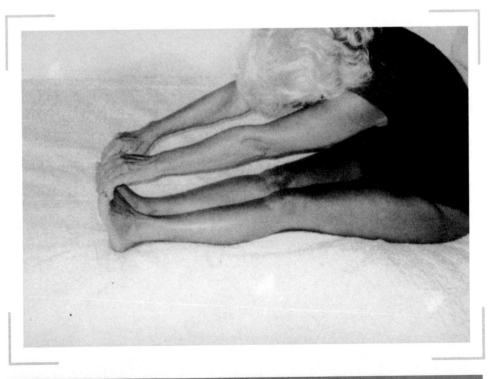

Exercise 59

Sit cross-legged or in any other position. Interlace your fingers, and press one hand down on the other, bending it, three times. Switch hands and the direction of the pressure. Repeat the exercise several times.

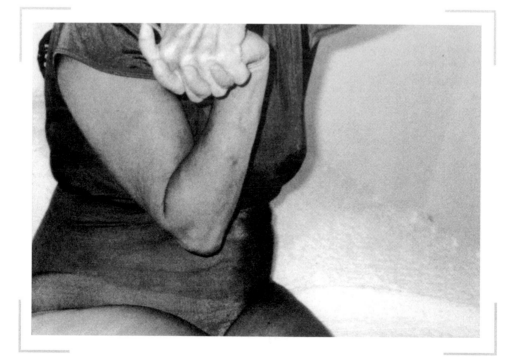

Exercise 60

Sit in the same position. Place your palms together, one hand pressing on the other and bending it, three times, pressing harder each time. Switch hands and repeat the exercise.

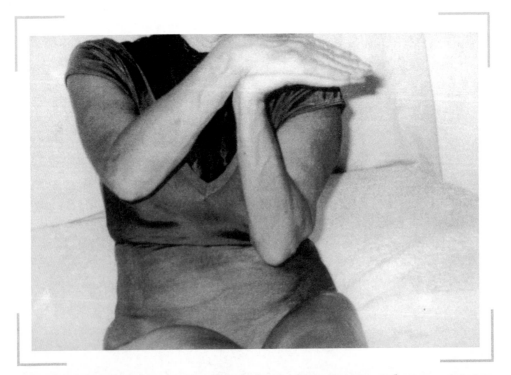

Exercise 61

Sit cross-legged or in any other way. (You can also stand.) Bend one arm backward, elbow upward, upper arm next to your head. Bend your other arm backward, elbow downward, near your waist, with the upper surface of your hand touching your back. Interlace the fingers of both hands and pull in opposite directions.

Switch hands and repeat the exercise.

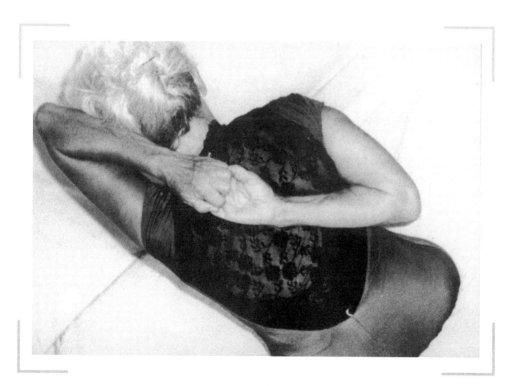

Exercise 62

Sit cross-legged or in any other position. (You can also lie on your stomach.) Apply pressure with both thumbs to the two treatment points in the region of the pelvis (see Introduction), while your hands support the muscles of your upper thighs. Each pressure takes five seconds, and is accompanied by rotation movements.

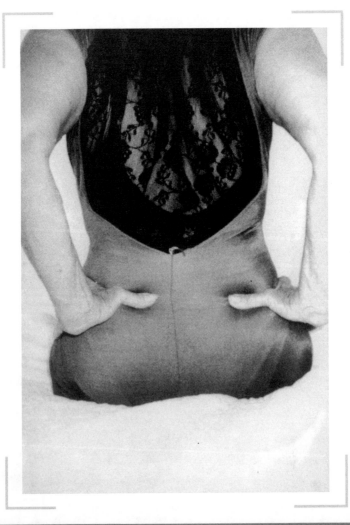

Exercise 63

Sit in the same position. Your elbows are far from your body. Apply T.P. along the two energy lines at the sides of the spine. Every pressure is accompanied by rotation movements, while lifting the muscle upward.

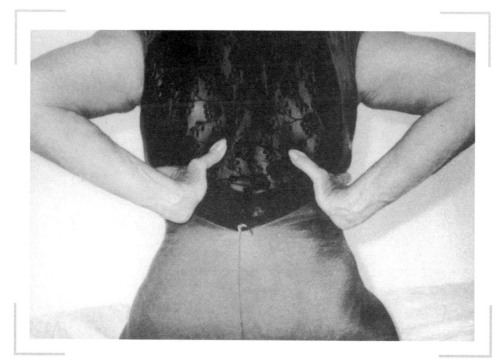

Exercise 64

Lie on your stomach. Grasp each leg in the region above your ankles with your hands, and bring your feet closer to your buttocks. Try and get your feet to touch your buttocks, and at the same time, lift your head as high as possible.

The result is that only your abdomen is on the floor. Your head, arms, and legs are in the air.

(This exercise requires a high level of pliancy; even if only parts of it are performed, that is also an achievement.)

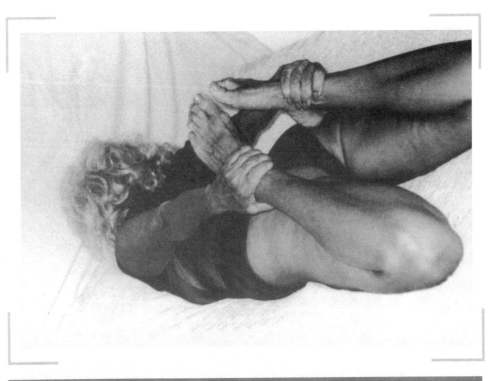

Exercise 65

Stand close to the wall. Place one hand on the wall, keeping your arm straight. Your foot on the same side is on the floor. Bend your other leg backward, and raise your ankle to your buttocks with your other hand. While holding the back of your bent leg, the other foot rises up above the floor, until only the pads of the toes are touching the floor.
Resume the position where your whole foot is on the floor, and repeat the exercise three times.
Repeat the exercise with the other foot, switching hands.

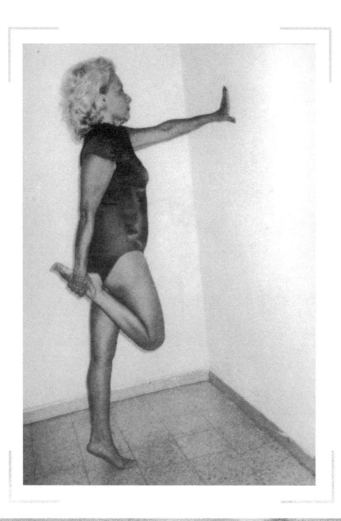

Exercise 66

Sit cross-legged or in any other position. Bend one arm backward, your hand holding the back of your neck. Support your forehead with your other hand, fingers close to each other.
Both hands apply counter pressure.
Switch hands and repeat the exercise.

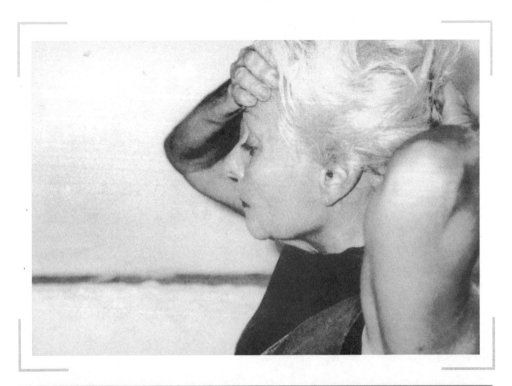

Exercise 67

Sit in the same position. Lift both arms above your head, your elbows as high as possible. Your interlaced fingers bend your head forward. One thumb is on top of the other, and they both apply press to all the points along the center line of the head (see Introduction).

Each point is pressed for five seconds by rotation movements.

The middle fingers can be used instead of the thumbs.

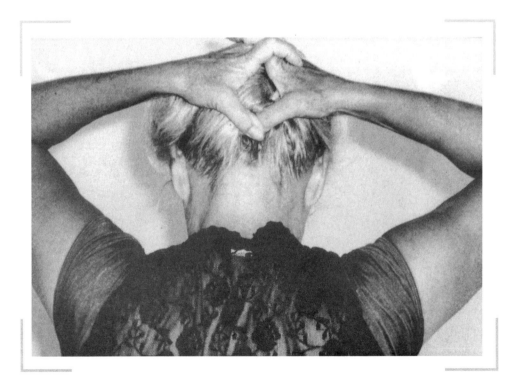

Exercise 68

Exercises for massaging the face begin with P.P. and turning movements
from the direction of the forehead to the chin and back. On the face,
there are several important treatment points (see Introduction).
Apply pressure to all these points with your thumbs and middle fingers
(whichever is more comfortable) for five seconds each, accompanied by
rotation movements.
The most important point is in the middle of the forehead - the third eye.

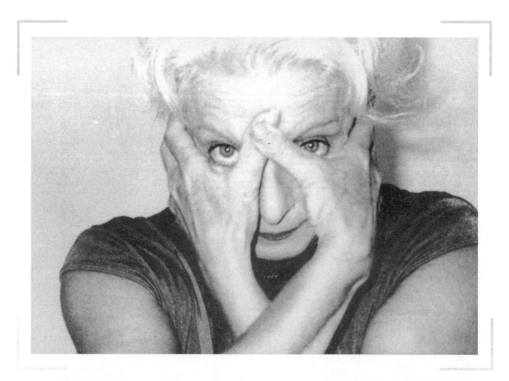

Exercise 69

Apply T.P. to your temples, your other fingers interlaced. Your hands support your chin while you apply pressure to the points on the temples. After the pressures, perform rotation movements.

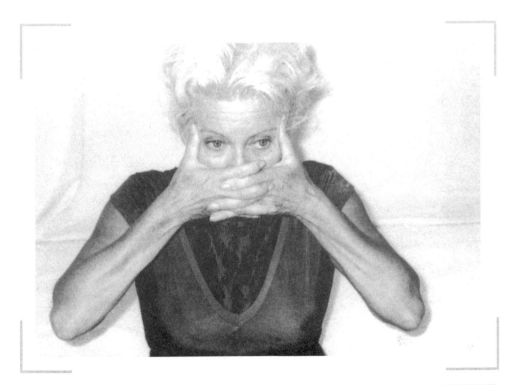

Exercise 70

You can perform exercise 69 when your hands, fingers interlaced, hold the top of your head, and the thumbs apply pressure to the temples.

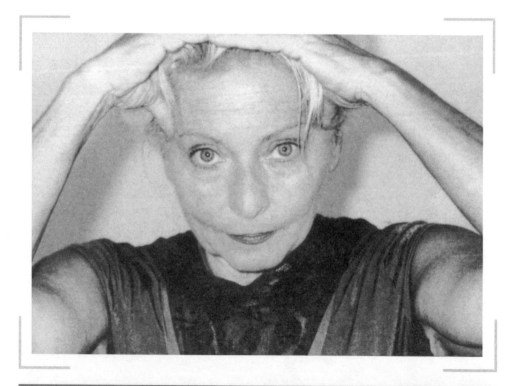

Exercise 71

Along the eyebrows, there are three treatment points (see Introduction). Apply thumb pressure to each point for five seconds, and then massage it with rotation movements. The pressure can be applied by the thumbs while the arms are straight, folded, or raised.

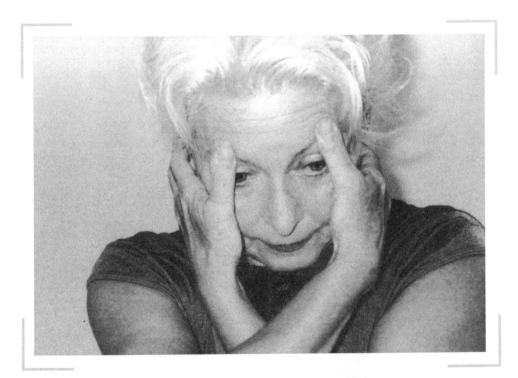

Exercise 72

In this exercise, specific pressure is applied to the tear ducts and the root of the nose for five seconds. You can apply the pressure with any finger that is comfortable for you.

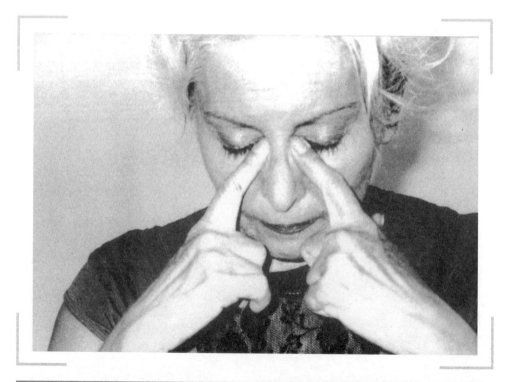

Exercise 73

On both sides of the nose, above the nostrils, there are two important treatment points. They are treated in exactly the same way as the other points in previous exercises: thumb pressure (or pressure with another finger), several times, 5-10 seconds on each point.

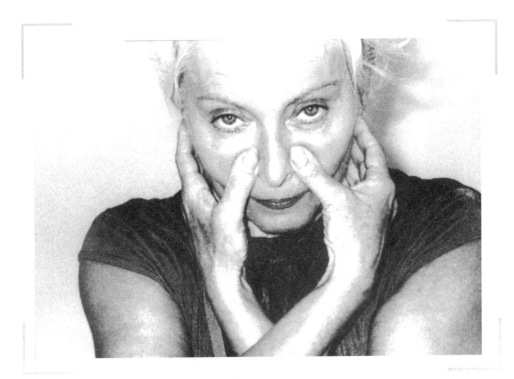

Exercise 74

You can perform this exercise with your middle fingers, with the other fingers supporting your head in several places in order to achieve stability during the application of pressure.

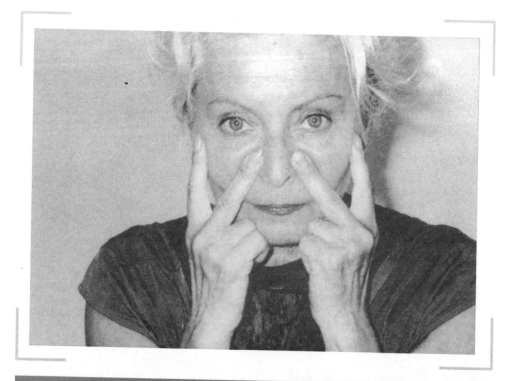

Exercise 75

In the middle of the chin, there is an extremely important treatment point. Pressure is applied to this point in a similar manner to previous exercises, with one thumb on top of the other, or with the middle finger. Apply pressure several times, for 5-10 seconds each time.

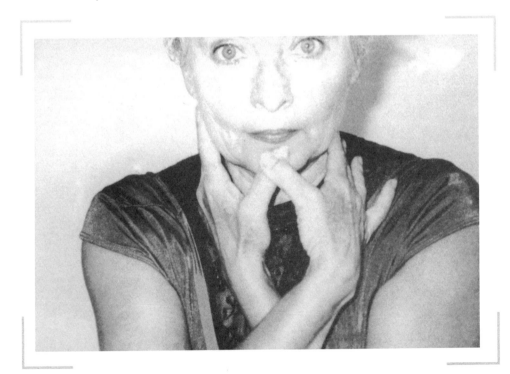

Exercise 76

When you have finished applying pressure and performing rotation movements on every single point, move your hands in stroking movements over your face. Rub your earlobes between your fingers, and pull them downward several times.

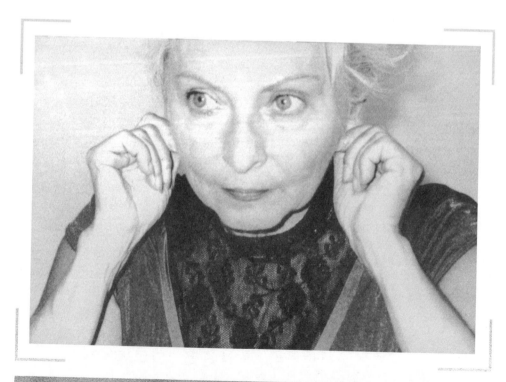

Exercise 77

At the end of the head and face massage, massage your scalp with the pads of your fingers for 30-60 seconds, using shampooing movements. The whole massage culminates in light stroking.

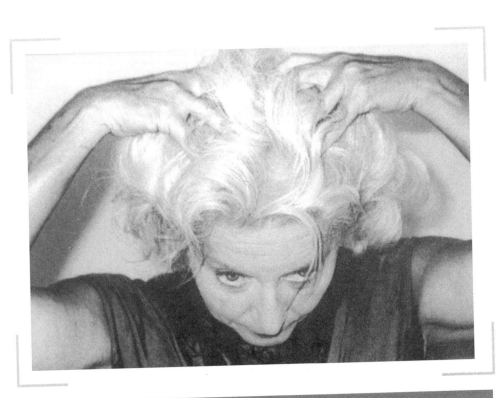

APPENDIX

Treatment of specific problems

The following information is only for the use of people who are qualified and have accumulated experience in Thai Massage Treatments, and that is because the patient who is suffering from local pains is especially sensitive to touch.

Treatment of lower back pains

When there are problems of lower back pains, the massage is performed as follows:

Massage of the abdomen (six points).
Massage of the legs (along inner energy line number 3).
Massage of the back.
Application of pressure to the treatment points (first T.P., then P.P.).

There are two main "reasons" for problems with lower back pains:

The muscles - for this reason, the massage is performed along the energy lines, between the muscles.

The spine - the pain is caused by the accumulation of calcium that presses on the nerve. The massage is performed along both sides of the spine.

Secondary reasons for back pains could be stomach, intestinal, or liver problems.

We start with five stages of massage:
Stretching, palm pressure, thumb pressure, palm pressure, and stretching.

Stage (a) - Abdominal massage

The patient lies on his back. The practitioner kneels.
The abdominal massage is applied to six points.
(See the list of treatment points on the abdomen in the Introduction.)

Stage (b) - Leg massage

The treatment begins with thumb pressure applied to point number 1, which is the join between the big toe and the second toe, above the upper surface of the foot. (See the list of treatment points on the leg in the Introduction.)

The pressures are applied in three stages: weak, medium, and strong. Each pressure is applied three times, for five seconds each time.

The massage continues with pressure on points number 2 and 3 along the outer energy line.

The thumbs apply all the pressure, and afterwards, rotation movements.

The exercise is repeated on the **other leg**.

Stage (c) - Back massage

The patient lies on his stomach. The massage is performed on the inner side of the legs, on points number 4, 5, 6, 7, 8A, 8B (see Introduction).

At the beginning of the massage, palm pressure is applied simultaneously to both legs, up to the waist. Afterward, pressure is applied to the above mentioned points by the thumbs, simultaneously on both legs. After every pressure, the thumbs perform rotation movements.

After massaging point number 8B, the massage is repeated for the sake of relaxation. Then palm pressures are applied to the back, up to the shoulders, and back again.

Stage (d) - Pressures

On point number 9, which is located on the tail bone, only rotation movements are applied.

On points number 10, 11, 12, which are located on the sides of the spine, palm pressures are applied three times, and afterward rotation movements by the thumbs.

On points number 13, 14, 15, 16, 17, thumb pressure is performed three times on each pair of points, from bottom to top, with each pressure lasting five seconds.

On point number 18, which is located behind the shoulder, and on point number 19, which is above the shoulder bone: thumb pressures are applied, and the exercise is completed with rotation movements.

The massage ends with palm pressures from the shoulders to the toes, according to the treatment points.

Stretching is not performed on the back. It can be performed on the legs.

Treatment of headaches and upper back pains

The stages of treatment:
Massage of the shoulders.
Massage of the back of the neck.
Massage of the back.
Acupressure.

The practitioner performs massage of the shoulders and nape (see the previous explanation), moves on to massage of the back along the two energy lines, and from there goes to the full massage of the head and neck. In the case of muscle cramps in the shoulder, massage of the arms must be applied, including twisting the arm backward and forward.

Treatment of neck pains and headaches

The stages of treatment:
Massage of the shoulders.
Massage of the nape.
Massage of the head.
Massage of the face.

The patient sits cross-legged. The practitioner kneels (or stands) behind him.

A. The massage of the shoulders is performed on both sides of the shoulder, including massage with the forearm.
B. The massage of the back of the neck is performed on the entire back of the head, followed by neck massage, both by palm pressure and by thumb pressure.
C. The massage of the head is performed along all the treatment points, and ends with shampooing movements.
D. The massage of the face is performed by pressing, stroking, and treatment of the massage points.

Comment: For every type of massage, see the Introduction and the first part of this book.

Treatment of knee pains

In the case of knee pain that is not caused by a fracture, the massage of the leg must be performed as follows:

Palm pressure.
Thumb pressure on the first outer and the third inner energy lines.
Blood stopping for 15-50 seconds.
Palm pressure for relaxation.

In the regions of the bones, the massage is performed by rotation movements.

On the leg, there are special treatment points to which special thumb pressures and acupressure must be applied.

The first treatment point is on the join between the foot and the leg, and it is located above the upper surface of the foot. Pressure must be applied by one thumb, while the other hand pushes the patient's leg backward while holding the toes. This exercise must be repeated several times. In this case, the most important energy line for treatment is the first outer energy line, especially for relaxation of the knee. Using the thumbs, the kneecap is pushed alternately up and down.

The second treatment point is located behind the kneecap, in the middle. When the patient lies on his side, thumb pressure (one on top of the other) must be applied to this point.

Bibliography

Brust, Harold: "The Art of Traditional Thai Massage." D.K. Editions Duang Kamol, 1994.

The Foundations of Shivago Komarpaj, "Thai Basic Massage." Chiang Mai, Thailand, 1995.

The author of the book, Beatrice Avraham, a qualified Thai massage practitioner from the Hospital for Alternative Medicine, Chiang Mai, Thailand, gives lectures and holds workshops (from the introduction for beginners, up to advanced studies for certification), and gives treatments and private lessons.

Thai massage combines touch, pressure, and stretching of the treatment points that are located along the energy lines in the human body.

The massage is performed in light and comfortable garments, and can be learned without the need for prior knowledge or special talents.

Every workshop includes a theoretical introduction (including videotapes), pair-work, and the study of self-massage.

The author can be contacted by e-mail or via the Internet:
thaiclin@netvision.net.il
www.thaiclinic.co.il